RECIPES FOR HEALTH

PMS

RECIPES FOR HEALTH

PMS

Over 100 recipes for overcoming premenstrual syndrome

JILL DAVIES
FOREWORD BY DR KATHARINA DALTON

Thorsons
An Imprint of HarperCollins*Publishers*

Thorsons
An Imprint of HarperCollins*Publishers*
77–85 Fulham Palace Road,
Hammersmith, London W6 8JB
1160 Battery Street,
San Francisco, California 94111–1213

First published by Thorsons as *Special Diet Cookbook:*
Premenstrual Syndrome 1991
This edition 1995
1 3 5 7 9 10 8 6 4 2

A catalogue record for this book
is available from the British Library

ISBN 0 7225 3140 0

Typeset by
Harper Phototypesetters Limited, Northampton, England
Printed in Great Britain by
HarperCollinsManufacturing Glasgow

Contents

Foreword   vii

Chapter 1   Facts about premenstrual syndrome   1
Chapter 2   Management of premenstrual syndrome   9
Chapter 3   Premenstrual syndrome and diet   17
Chapter 4   Breakfasts   35
Chapter 5   Between-meal snacks   50
Chapter 6   Light meals   86
Chapter 7   Main meals   117
             Starters   117
             Main dishes   133
             Carbohydrate 'rich' dishes   158
             Vegetables and salads   168
             Sweets   182
Chapter 8   Emergency snacks   191

Further Reading   199
Useful Addresses   200
General Index   201
Recipe Index   203

Foreword

AT LAST! A cookbook for the sufferer of premenstrual syndrome (PMS) written by a nutritionalist who understands the cause and pathology of premenstrual syndrome. As a consequence she recognizes the importance for sufferers of the essential nutritional requirement of eating small snacks of starchy food every three hours in addition to a normal healthy diet. She has selected her recipes accordingly. I am delighted with the result.

Premenstrual syndrome is the presence of recurrent symptoms before menstruation with complete absence of symptoms after menstruation. Those suffering from PMS have a special problem relating to their diet, which is of importance regardless of any medication they are receiving. Their problem is that they need to avoid a drop in their blood sugar level for this sparks off a release of adrenalin, which in turn prevents the progesterone receptors in the cells binding to molecules of progesterone. This recognition of progesterone receptors is quite recent and is seen as a breakthrough in our understanding of the action of progesterone. It has shed a new light on the cause of premenstrual syndrome and postnatal depression.

The normal task of the progesterone receptors is to transport the molecules of progesterone into the nucleus of cells, where progesterone can be converted and used. So without the progesterone receptors working it does not matter how much progesterone there is in the blood, for the cells cannot utilize it. Avoidance of a drop in the blood sugar is best achieved by eating throughout the entire month small portions of starchy foods (complex carbohydrates) every three hours, and always within one hour of rising and one hour of retiring. In short it is recommended that she changes to a nibbling diet of six snacks daily instead of the more conventional one or two big meals each day.

It is appreciated that the PMS sufferer also needs a good healthy diet, and so the nutritional significance of sugar, complex carbohydrates, fats, salt, alcohol and caffeine is discussed. All too often the PMS sufferer is not alone, but part of a family or community. The dietary suggestions given in this book are suitable for all who aim at a healthy, nutritious diet, and the many interesting recipes can be enjoyed by the whole family.

It is now appreciated that PMS is due to the problem of the progesterone receptors in the cells which manifest themselves when the progesterone level in the blood is raised, such as during those days from ovulation to menstruation. If PMS sufferers, or indeed anyone, are having a good healthy diet, then there is no need for them to require nutritional supplements. During the menstrual cycle there is no evidence of a fluctuation in the blood level of vitamin B_6 (pyridoxine), magnesium, zinc or any vitamin or minerals, and no evidence that these are required by PMS sufferers any more than by non-suffering women or men.

Recent surveys have shown that as many as 30 per cent of severe PMS sufferers can be helped by the three-hourly starch régime alone, without the need of medication. Many, who have benefitted, have asked me for a cookbook. This is one I will now be able to recommend with confidence.

Dr Katharina Dalton
March 1991

Facts about Premenstrual Syndrome

HOW MANY GIRLS AND WOMEN SUFFER FROM PREMENSTRUAL SYNDROME?

Premenstrual syndrome (PMS) is a common condition which affects girls and women during their reproductive years. It can occur at any time between *the onset of monthly periods* and *the change of life*. Opinion varies on how common it is. It is generally agreed that about 30 to 40 per cent of all women are affected with some symptoms of PMS, and 5 to 10 per cent are severely affected. Whatever the precise incidence, PMS is undoubtedly a problem for a significant number of girls and women.

WHAT ARE THE SYMPTOMS OF PMS?

About 150 different symptoms have been identified. A summary of the major ones is given in Table 1, overleaf.

TABLE 1 MAJOR SYMPTOMS OF PMS

Physical	Psychological
• Back pain, sore joints	• Anxiety
• Breast tenderness, soreness	• Aggression
• Changes in sex drive	• Crying for no apparent reason
• Clumsiness	• Depression
• Food cravings – for example, sweet or salty foods	• Difficulty in concentrating, forgetfulness, confusion
• Headaches, migraine	• Fatigue and loss of energy
• Skin problems	• Irritability
• Sore throat, nasal catarrh, styes	• Loss of confidence
• Weight gain, feeling bloated, especially in the abdomen	• Mood swings
	• Tension

The symptoms, however, are only part of the story, what is particularly important is the time when they occur. This is very aptly summed up by the Dalton Society definition of PMS: 'the recurrence of symptoms before menstruation with complete ABSENCE of symptoms after menstruation'. The symptoms usually start 1 to 14 days before the beginning of the period, and relief usually occurs within the first two days of the onset of the period. The symptoms recur every month before menstruation and disappear shortly after menstruation begins.

WHO SUFFERS FROM PMS?

It is not just those who have been diagnosed as having PMS who suffer. Some of the symptoms put a great deal of strain on others close to them. Adolescents, for example, who suffer from PMS can become very awkward and this puts a strain on family life. PMS can have disastrous consequences in relationships: marriages have even broken up as a result of the condition. Men have claimed that they 'can't do anything right' and, in extreme cases, women have become impossible to live with. Some women have actually physically attacked their partners. Children can also suffer from the effects of living with a PMS sufferer, and some develop ailments, such as coughs, runny noses, vomiting and temper tantrums. Even more serious, some children become the victims of child battering. Industry also suffers – the days off work, in Britain, resulting from PMS amount to 3 per cent of the wage bill, and efficiency decreases even when the sufferer soldiers on.

To find out if you have PMS, keep a record of your symptoms, showing actual dates and timing of bleeding. A practical way to do this is to keep a chart like the one shown on page 4. Such a record is critical in diagnosing PMS. In medical circles it is agreed that the presence of symptoms pre-menstrually, and their absence post-menstrually, is the key to diagnosis. This record-keeping may seem rather tedious, but it is worth taking care over the charting as this will enable your GP to make an accurate diagnosis.

HOW DO YOU KNOW
IF YOU HAVE PMS?

FIGURE 1 PMS RECORD CHART

	J	F	M	A	M	J	J	A	S	O	N	D
1												
2												
3												
4												
5												
6												
7												
8												
9												
10												
11												
12												
13												
14												
15												
16												
17												
18												
19												
20												
21												
22												
23												
24												

PMS

	J	F	M	A	M	J	J	A	S	O	N	D
25												
26												
27												
28												
29												
30												
31												

By kind permission of PMS Help
P.O. Box 160, St Albans, Herts AL1 4UQ

Mark on this chart the days of menstruation with an **M** and the days of your **three priority symptoms** with a symbol. For example:

B = breast tenderness
H = headache
X = awful day
M = menstruation

Do not be put off by any doctor who feels 'that PMS does not exist, or that, if it does, it is in the mind of the distraught woman . . .' If your doctor is unsympathetic, find and consult another health professional. Ask your local pharmacist, he usually knows the likes and dislikes of local doctors.

WHAT CAUSES PMS?

'There used to be no precise explanation about the cause of PMS'. The following gives a general insight into the nature of the problem so that the different strategies for treating the condition (see pages 9–16) will be more meaningful.

Many people feel that PMS is due to an hormonal imbalance (hormones are chemical messengers). It is sometimes described as a 'progesterone-responsive disease' because individually-tailored treatment with the hormone, progesterone, has proved to be helpful in relieving the symptoms; (progesterone is made in the ovaries which are almond shaped and positioned on either side of the pelvis).

Progesterone serves a number of different functions in the body, for example, the preparation of the uterus (womb) before fertilization. It also plays an important role in the regulation of blood glucose (the sugar found in blood) commonly referred to as blood sugar, and it is this aspect which is particularly relevant to PMS. However, in order to understand the events as they apply to PMS, it is first necessary to know a little about the blood sugar regulating mechanisms.

Blood sugar levels are influenced by different factors. For example, after a carbohydrate-rich meal, the sugar level will rise; conversely, after starvation, the sugar level will fall. Various hormones play a part in maintaining blood sugar levels; perhaps the best known of these is insulin which is produced in the pancreas (some of this gland lies behind the stomach, to the left side, and part is encircled by the duodenum). Should the level of blood sugar become too high, as it can in diabetes, the *upper regulating mechanism* comes into action, there is a spurt of insulin and the excess sugar escapes in urine via the kidneys. Conversely, should the level of blood sugar fall drastically, as it can in starvation, the *lower regulating mechanism* may come into action. When this happens, adrenalin, a hormone produced by the adrenal glands, surges into the blood and causes some of the body cells to release sugar (the adrenal glands lie at the upper end of the kidneys).

Getting back to progesterone, and remembering that PMS is a progesterone-responsive disease, it should be noted that progesterone plays a role in the *lower regulating mechanism*. If the amount of progesterone is insufficient, the baseline for the lower level of blood sugar is raised. This means that the *lower regulating mechanism* comes into action earlier and surges of adrenalin occur sooner. This is shown in Figure 2, p. 8.

At face value, adrenalin to the rescue sounds fine because the lowered blood sugar is raised. However, the withdrawal of sugar from the body cells tends to result in waterlogging of the cells, and fluid retention is a well-known feature of PMS. Furthermore, the adrenalin accumulates in the body causing a number of side effects, all of which are characteristic of PMS. These may include: unexpected aggression; sudden loss of control; migraine; irritability; panic attacks; crying; palpitations and epilepsy. Katharina Dalton explains this process in her writing on PMS: 'Progesterone receptors, which are present in the cells, normally transfer molecules of progesterone into the cell and across the nuclear wall to the nucleus, where the progesterone molecule is metabolised and used. If adrenalin is present the progesterone receptor will not transport molecules of progesterone.'

A hormone called prolactin, which is produced in the pituitary gland, is of interest in the story (the pituitary gland lies in the skull at the base of the brain). A high level of prolactin can produce PMS-like symptoms, which are present throughout the cycle, but not PMS symptoms which are limited to the premenstruum and absent in the postmenstruum. However, most PMS sufferers have 'normal' levels of prolactin and it has been suggested that lack of a particular hormone-like substance, called prostaglandin E, can cause hypersensitivity to 'normal' prolactin levels. The prostaglandins are derived from essential fatty acids in the diet. Lack of prostaglandin E can produce an hormonal imbalance.

FIGURE 2 BLOOD SUGAR AND PMS

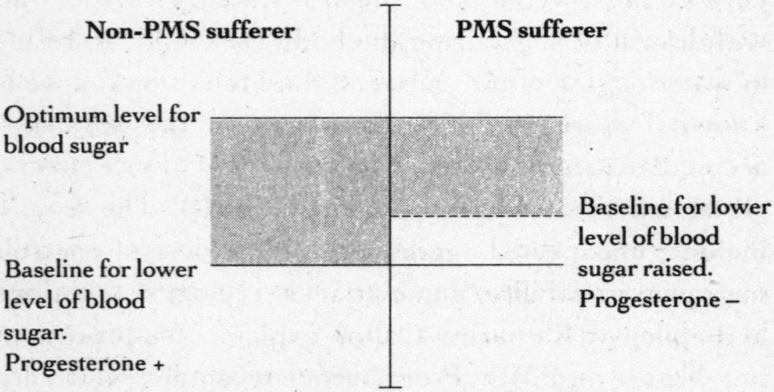

Diagram adapted from ideas presented in *Once a Month* by K. Dalton, published by Fontana (1987)

Management of Premenstrual Syndrome

DIETARY MANAGEMENT OF PMS

Diet is a key issue in the management of PMS.

Carbohydrate

Foods rich in *starch* are very important in the treatment of PMS. 'Starchy' foods come under the umbrella of carbo-hydrates and include bread, pasta and rice. Starch is made up of hundreds or even thousands of molecules. Starch has an important role to play in PMS as it causes a gradual rise in blood sugar level and a gradual fall. If foods rich in starch are not highly refined for example wholemeal (wholewheat) bread as opposed to white bread they are useful sources of dietary fibre (roughage) or what nutritionists call *non-starch polysaccharides*. These foods are described as being rich in *complex carbohydrates*.

Sugars also come under the heading of carbohydrate but their structure is much simpler. Sugars are made up of one or two molecules only. Foods rich in sugars include jam, sweets and chocolate. Sugar causes a sudden rise in blood sugar level and a rapid drop and is not the solution to the low blood sugar levels associated with PMS.

What about those foods which contain starch and sugar? For example cakes and biscuits include flour and sugar in their recipes. As far as PMS is concerned the mixture is fine because although the sugar will cause a rapid rise, the starch will ensure a more gradual drop in blood sugar level. However in the context of healthy eating it is advisable to wean yourself away from the 'sweet tooth syndrome'.

Meal Spacing

Throughout the month the timing of meals is a critical issue. It is important to eat small portions of food rich in complex carbohydrate at *3-hourly intervals* during the day. Such foods should also be eaten within 1 hour of rising and 1 hour of sleeping. Depending upon physical activity it may be necessary to have extra portions to allow for the additional energy expenditure. Following this régime (see pp. 29–32) the blood sugar levels should be maintained.

HORMONE THERAPY

The effectiveness of progesterone therapy is very well documented by Dr Katharina Dalton (see Further Reading list p. 199). But it is now appreciated that progesterone therapy is ineffective if the blood sugar level drops.

Progesterone Suppositories and Pessaries

Small pellets of wax, containing progesterone, may be prescribed. These are inserted in the vagina or the rectum. Absorption rates vary, so dosage needs to be carefully monitored. The usual time for using the pellets is mid-cycle (ovulation) until the beginning of the menstrual flow.

Note of caution: any thrush infections in both the patient and her partner need to be cleared up before progesterone pessaries are used as these can exacerbate the condition.

Progesterone Injections

These are ideal for the small percentage of women who are unable to absorb progesterone effectively through the vagina or rectum. The advantage of this treatment is that the rate of absorption is highly efficient and good for crisis situations.

Progesterone Implants

This form of therapy is generally suitable for women who have responded well to progesterone suppositories, pessaries or injections. The implant lasts for an average of three to four months, although it can last much longer. Implants are not ideal for some people, and expert advice is important. One possible side effect of implants is inflammation at the implant site.

Progestogens

Synthetic hormones, called progestogens, may be prescribed. Their use, however, for managing PMS is controversial. As Dr Katharina Dalton points out: 'There are many differences between progesterone and the various progestogens, but unfortunately there are still some doctors who do not realize this'. If you are particularly interested in this treatment, see Further Reading list, page 199.

PHARMACOLOGICAL PREPARATIONS

Bromocriptine

This drug works by suppressing the secretion of prolactin by the pituitary gland. It may be of benefit in reducing bloatedness, breast discomfort and lethargy in those patients with a raised prolactin level. Dosage needs to be carefully monitored because this drug is very powerful. Side effects may include dizziness, nausea, vomiting, headaches, constipation and a fall in blood pressure.

Diuretics

Treatment for PMS based on diuretics is limited. Any benefits are associated with water-retention symptoms only: for example, weight gain, bloatedness and swollen ankles. Moreover, the benefits are short term. Diuretics can become addictive and long-term usage may cause a lowering of the blood potassium level.

Anti-Depressants

Treatment with anti-depressant drugs has not had a high success rate. The choice of drug needs to be carefully considered. One particular group of anti-depressant drugs has been associated with a reduction of blood levels of progesterone, that symptoms, such as bloatedness and lethargy, may actually worsen. Another drawback is that anti-depressants are addictive and can cause dependency.

Tranquillizers

Surprisingly some doctors prescribe tranquillizers for PMS. Tranquillizers may relieve irritability and violent outbursts, but they can also cause depression and tiredness. The use of this type of drug for PMS is generally frowned upon and has no place in sound management of the condition.

NUTRITIONAL SUPPLEMENTS

Vitamin B₆ (Pyridoxine)

The value of this form of treatment in controlling PMS is under debate and there is no evidence from well controlled clinical tests that it is effective. On the contrary, there is alarming evidence that as many as 60 per cent of those taking vitamin B_6 in doses of around 25mg a day suffer nervous contraindications often typical of the characteristics of PMS itself, such as head aches, tiredness, depression, irritability and bloatedness. Other symptoms of overdose which may develop later are muscle weakness and pins and needles in the face, arms and legs. Since the prescribed dose of vitamin B_6 for PMS is usually 100–200mg/day for up to 3 months the danger of overdose needs to be borne in mind.

There are some studies which claim its virtues however, particularly in relieving breast discomfort. The Reference Nutrient Intake (RNI) for vitamin B_6 is around 1.0–1.2mg/day and a mixed diet based on healthy eating guidelines will provide this, so that a vitamin supplement is unnecessary. Useful sources include liver, meat, eggs and vegetables.

Evening Primrose Oil

The use of evening primrose oil is based on the theory that PMS is the result of a deficiency of the hormone-like substance prostaglandin E_1. The normal metabolic pathway, involved in the production of prostaglandin E_1, begins with essential fatty acids in the diet. Evening primrose oil offers a short-cut approach in this sequence. The treatment has been associated with mild-to-moderate benefit for PMS sufferers with breast pain, though recent medical studies have shown that this is solely a placebo effect and as a consequence it is not usually available on prescription.

The prescribed dosage of evening primrose oil is around 6x500mg/day throughout the menstrual cycle for two months. After this it is usually reduced to about half this amount. It is expensive, and the gelatin coating of the commonly available form, *Efamol*, precludes vegetarians

from its use. To ensure adequate amounts of prostaglandin E_1, it is prudent to make any necessary adjust-
ments to diet. For this purpose, include a supply of
vegetable oils, such as sunflower, safflower and corn oil,
and eat a healthy mixed diet. This should supply
adequate amounts of the nutrients involved in the metabolic sequence.

PSYCHOTHERAPY

This treatment can give considerable benefit in certain
circumstances: for example, if there are underlying
personal or domestic problems. Therapy of this type can
be provided by a general practitioner or by referral to a
psychotherapist.

CHANGES TO LIFESTYLE

A few changes to lifestyle may help PMS sufferers.
Perhaps this is the time to take stock of certain issues.
Ask yourself the following questions:

1. Do you get a 'good' night's sleep?
2. Do you allow time for regular physical exercise?
3. Do you take time to relax? (This is especially
   important in the second part of the menstrual cycle.)
4. Do you always eat some starchy food within one hour
   of waking and one hour of retiring?
5. Do you smoke?
6. Are you taking oral contraceptives?

7. Do you drink alcohol excessively or at all during the premenstrual phase?
8. Do you ever go longer than three hours without a nibble of starchy food?

If you answered 'yes' to the first four questions and 'no' to the last four, you have decreased your chances of suffering from PMS. If not, then take stock.

3

Premenstrual Syndrome and Diet

FOODS FOR THOUGHT

Sugar

Sugar is often described as 'empty calories' as it provides little more than energy. High intakes may be associated with obesity and dental caries. Healthy eating guidelines recommend a reduction in the amount of sugar that we eat. This is good advice for all of us, but excellent advice for PMS sufferers. To recap on this very important point, sugar causes a rapid rise and fall in blood sugar levels (see page 10). To reduce the amount of sugar you eat you can:

Familiarize yourself with the names of different types of sugar. For example: cane syrup, dextrose, honey, lactose, malt extract, maple syrup, glucose syrup and sucrose. Then, to be sure to read food labels carefully and avoid foods which contain these. Look for statements, such as 'without added sugar' and opt for these foods in preference to sugar-containing counterparts. For example, use fruit canned in its own juice rather than in sugar syrup.

Breakfast Cereal

When deciding which cereal to have, avoid those with sugary coatings, and remember not to ruin the good intention by sprinkling with sugar. Chopped fresh or dried fruit can be used to enhance the sweetness of breakfast cereals.

Jam

As a change from traditional jam, try the delicious range of low-sugar jams, or, better still, fruit spreads.

'Convenience' Foods

Sauces often contain sugar. So, why not prepare your own? Kitchen gadgets, such as liquidizers (blenders), food processors and microwave ovens, can make this a speedy procedure.

Cakes and Biscuits

These can easily be made using little or no sugar simply by making use of fresh and dried fruit, and vegetables, such as carrots.

Adding Sugar or Honey to Drinks

Break the habit. In terms of healthy eating, it is advisable to lose your 'sweet tooth', and to remember that sugary drinks throughout the day will hinder the achievement of this goal.

Between Meal Snacks

These can greatly increase sugar intake if due care and

attention are not exercised. Consider, instead, savoury foods or specially-formulated low-sugar recipes, see the recipe section, p. 50, as a healthy alternative for all the family.

Sweets

If you really can't live without a pudding as an end to a main meal, by all means have one. However, choose specially-formulated low-sugar recipes as mentioned above. Ideally, though, try leaving puddings off the menu.

FAT

Most people living in the UK and Westernized society eat much more fat than they need. A reduction in fat, particularly saturated fat (the fat that is generally solid at room temperature) is wise. High intakes of saturated fat are associated with an increase in blood levels of cholesterol, a well known risk factor in coronary heart disease. To help in this process some of the saturated fat can be replaced with unsaturated fat (the fat which is usually liquid at room temperature). This obviously has relevance to the prostaglandin PMS theory (see p. 8) as well as being sensible in terms of healthy eating. To cut down on the amount of fat in your diet:

- Eat bread, crispbread and crackers without a spreading of fat. If you use interesting toppings such as the Lentil Pâté on page 121 the fat will not be missed. Alternatively, try a low-fat spread.

- Refrain from serving jacket potatoes and vegetables with the infamous knob of butter. Use, instead, yogurt dressings and liberal sprinklings of freshly-chopped herbs.
- Don't flood your food with fat-based sauces, such as gravy, white sauces, and parsley sauce. Substitute skimmed milk for whole milk to make low-fat versions of these products.
- When meat is on the menu, choose lean cuts; go for 'quality' mince or make your own, using lean meat; opt for low-fat rather than full-fat sausages; have chicken, but remember not to eat the skin as this is fatty; and choose white meat in preference to brown, as this is lower in fat content. Meat dishes, based on pastry, should be a thing of the past; and grill rather than fry meat.
- Say farewell to whole milk. This is approximately 4 per cent fat. Use semi-skimmed, low fat or skimmed milks which are 1.5 to 1.8 per cent and less than 0.3 per cent fat respectively.
- Remember that cheese varies enormously in fat content. Try some of the specially manufactured low-fat varieties which are less than half the fat of their traditional counterparts. When making cheese dishes, use really strongly flavoured cheeses, such as Parmesan and 'extra' mature Cheddar, so that you can use less cheese.
- Instead of using cream, choose alternatives, such as Dream Topping, made up with semi-skimmed, low-fat or skimmed milk. Try fromage frais and low-fat

varieties of yogurt instead of cream.

- Be conscious of the so called *hidden fats* in cakes, pastries and biscuits. You may be better off going for buns, sweetened breads, scones and certain types of cake.
- When fried foods are on the menu, keep the fat content to the minimum: always cook the food at the recommended temperature for frying. If you really can't live without fried food, buy a frying thermometer. Seal burgers with a coating of egg and crumbs to prevent fat absorption during cooking; drain fried foods on kitchen paper (paper towels) as soon as the food is cooked.

COMPLEX CARBOHYDRATE FOODS

To compensate for the reduction in sugar and fat intakes eat more complex carbohydrate – 'starchy foods, fibre and all'. This is particularly helpful for PMS sufferers.

To recap: starchy foods cause the blood sugar levels to rise and fall gradually. Increasing complex carbohydrate at the expense of fat will cause a fall in energy intake. This is because 1g of the former yields 3.75 Kcals and 1g of the latter 9Kcals. Complex carbohydrate in contrast to simple sugars also contains useful amounts of dietary fibre and fibre is often described as an 'obstacle to energy intake'. Therefore do not get anxious about calories! If you are particularly interested in this aspect see further reading p. 199, (*Food: The Definitive Guide*). The fibre that is present is a welcome dietary asset for PMS sufferers who are constipated. Moreover, most of us living in the Western World have a tendency to eat too little dietary fibre, 13g/day when, in fact, most people need 18g/day.

To increase the amount of complex carbohydrate in your diet:

• Choose unrefined foods in preference to refined. Examples of these are shown in Table 2, below.

TABLE 2 UNREFINED CARBOHYDRATE-RICH FOODS VERSUS REFINED CARBOHYDRATE

	Dietary fibre %	
Food	Unrefined	Refined
Bread wholemeal (wholewheat)	5.8	
White		1.5
Rice: cooked brown	0.8	
white		0.2
Pasta: cooked wholemeal (wholewheat)	3.5	
white		1.2

Taken from 'cereals and products', the third supplement to McCance & Widdowson's *The Composition of Foods* (4th edition) by B. Holland, I.D. Unwin and D.H. Buss, published by the Royal Society of Chemistry 1988.

- When deciding the focal point of meals, consider using pulses instead of meat, fish, eggs and cheese. Canned pulses, such as red kidney beans, chickpeas and, of course, baked beans are readily available. If you have a pressure cooker you can prepare your own pulses economically using dried varieties. The recipe section (see p. 107) gives lots of enjoyable ways to use pulses.
- Don't just serve bread as 'bread' or toast. Use it creatively in recipes. It can be used as a filler in a burger and loaf mixtures; as a coating, especially for fried food (see p. 21); to make a crunchy topping for savoury and sweet dishes; as a thickening agent in soups and sauces; as a basis for puddings; and, last but not least, for stuffings. Bread has certainly crept into many of the recipes in this book. Menopausal women may be concerned about the lower calcium content and higher phytate and dietary fibre content of wholemeal (wholewheat) bread in contrast to white bread. Phytate and fibre both hinder the absorption of calcium. However, this should not pose a problem if foods rich in calcium are eaten (see further reading p. 199, *Food: The Definitive Guide*). Generally dairy foods including milk, yogurt and cheese and fish eaten with bones are a useful source of calcium.
- Similarly, make use of breakfast cereals in recipes. The high-fibre varieties, such as All-Bran, are excellent in loaves and cakes, and crumbled up cereals can be used as coatings and toppings.
- When preparing vegetables try to leave outer skins

on. Do not over-cook, aim at a crunchy or, at least, a firm texture.

- In the case of fruit, you will 'obviously' have to discard some skins, for example banana and pineapple. But fruit such as apples, pears and plums can be left intact. Leaving skins on adds considerably to the fibre content of the diet.

A note of caution: although fresh fruit is delicious on its own, it is not a substitute for a meal or between meal snack for PMS sufferers

Salt

In the past those with PMS symptoms associated with fluid retention were advised to cut down their intake of salt. (It is now known that the fluid retention is related to the low blood sugar level, however, so a reduction in salt is not now vital.) However, most people in the UK consume about four times the amount of salt required. To cut down:

- Look at food labels and choose foods which state: 'without added salt'.
- Limit your intake of foods preserved with salt, for example bacon and kippers.
- Avoid adding salt when cooking vegetables, rice and pasta.
- Note that flavourings, such as garlic salt and celery salt, are salt-based. Use fresh garlic or fresh celery instead.

- Stop putting the salt cellar out at meal times – 'out of sight out of mind'.
- Try a substitute, such as low sodium and high-potassium salts.

Water

The body needs a regular supply of water, which comes in the form of food and drink, and is also obtained as a result of metabolic processes. If you suffer from fluid retention, however, you may need to cut down on your liquid intake. But, bearing in mind that some water is essential to the body's needs, aim at about 1140ml/40 fl oz/5 cups daily.

Alcoholic Drinks

PMS sufferers are advised to be cautious about intakes of alcohol. The effects of alcohol are particularly felt during the pre-menstruum. Some doctors advise PMS patients to abstain from alcohol altogether at this stage of the cycle. To reduce the amount of alcohol in your diet:

- Designate a few days each week, especially when you are premenstrual, 'alcohol free', and compensate with refreshing, unsugared alternatives.
- Despite the temptation after a hard day, avoid drinking on your own.
- Alternate alcoholic drinks with non-alcoholic drinks, and for half-wine and mineral or soda water drinks.

Caffeinated Beverages

Caffeine is found in drinks, such as tea, coffee, cocoa and cola-type beverages. Caffeine is a stimulant. It will trigger PMS-like symptoms throughout the month such as tension, irritability, anxiety or mood swings. It will cause increased alertness, but never 'fatigue'! To cut down on caffeine intake:

- Make your drinks, such as tea and coffee, much more diluted than usual.
- Only have one cup of tea and one cup of coffee daily.
- Try some of the exciting alternatives, such as herbal teas and decaffeinated coffee.

A NEW PATTERN OF EATING

If you have PMS, three meals a day are not enough. In order to keep your blood sugar from falling to danger levels you need to eat an average of six meals a day at three-hourly intervals:

1. Breakfast.
2. Between-meal-snack.
3. Midday meal.
4. Between-meal-snack.
5. Evening meal.
6. Between-meal-snack.

TABLE 3: DIETARY REFERENCE VALUES FOR ENERGY

Group	Age (years)	Estimated Average Requirement (Kcals/day)
Girls	11–14	1845
	15–18	2110
Women	19–50	1940

Taken from 'Dietary Reference Values for Food Energy and Nutrients for the United Kingdom. Department of Health'. Published by HMSO, 1991.

Your immediate reaction will probably be what about the calories? You are right to be concerned; but there are solutions to the problem. You could, for example, simply eat half your usual portion size for breakfast, midday and evening meals and eat crispbreads and crackers between meals. If you have a sandwich-type meal, you could eat half your usual portion for the meal, and eat the remaining half as a between meal snack. On the other hand, you could use the delicious recipes in this book and not be in excess of the Estimated Average Requirement for Energy (see Table 3 above). All the main meal recipes in this book indicate that PMS sufferers should have a half portion.

The recipes have been very carefully formulated and the portion size has been adjusted to ensure that, whilst your blood sugar is never allowed to fall to danger levels, your energy intake will not escalate. See the suggested seven-day eating plan Table 4, pp. 29–32. This allows you flexibility with regard to drinks and additional between meal snacks should you have an unusually long day, just fancy a 'bit extra' at a given meal or engage in vigorous energy expenditure!

The eating plan also allows for emergency situations. For example you may be stuck in a traffic jam, the train may break down, or you may have to stay late at work. In such circumstances, you may find that the three-hourly interval without food is running out of time. If this is the case, you will need to have a supply of 'emergency measures' (see p. 191).

The seven-day eating plan is merely a guide. Using the recipes in this book will allow you to come up with a number of permutations on the same theme. When planning breakfast, midday and evening meals, be sure to include foods from the groups shown in Figure 3. If you do this, you will ensure a healthy mixture. Remember that it is much easier to plan your meals around foods than around nutrients. If you keep to this simple rule you should not lack the essential nutrients.

FIGURE 3 CHOOSE FOODS FROM THESE GROUPS

Food Group	Example
'Protein rich'	Meat, poultry, fish, eggs, milk, cheese, pulses, nuts
Cereals	Bread, crispbread, pasta, rice, breakfast cereals
Fruit and vegetables	Oranges, apples, bananas, carrots, cauliflower, potatoes

TABLE 4 TYPICAL SEVEN-DAY EATING PLAN SHOWING ENERGY VALUES (PER MEAL/DAY)

Day	Breakfast	Between meal snack	Light meal
Monday	1 glass unsweetened fruit juice. Crunchy brek with low-fat plain yogurt. (335)	1 slice stilton loaf. (195)	1 wholemeal/ wholewheat pitta pocket filled with tuna, cucumber and yogurt. 1 orange (355)
Tuesday	1 glass unsweetened fruit juice. 2 bran muffins with poly- unsaturated margarine. (305)	1 baked bean burger. (140)	Cheese and mushroom pâté, wholemeal/ wholewheat toast. 1 apple. (210)
Wednesday	1 glass unsweetened fruit juice. Herring in apple and oatmeal. (315)	1 slice cheesy loaf. (125)	1 Scotch egg, tabbouleh, mushroom salad. Bunch of grapes. (455)
Thursday	1 glass unsweetened fruit juice. Muesli. (435)	Pot-snack: potato salad and ham. (125)	2 salmon fish cakes, tomato and basil salad. 1 banana. (365)

Between meal snack	Main meal	Between meal snack	Total Kcals
1 slice carrot and hazelnut cake.	Potato dip. Lamb with dried fruit, couscous, fruity carrot salad. Yogurt treat.	2 oaty biscuits/ cookies.	
(120)	(465)	(130)	1600
1 potato and parsnip cake.	Lentil soup. Fish pie, green salad with mint, tomato and basil salad. Apple crunch.	2 digestive biscuits/Graham crackers.	
(120)	(480)	(130)	1385
Garlic bites.	Avocado with fruit. Chilli-con-carne, vegetable rice, minty cucumber salad. Banana surprise.	1 slice banana and walnut/English walnut cake.	
(110)	(450)	(215)	1695
1 potato and spinach cake	Lentil pâté, wholemeal/ wholewheat toast. Toad in the hole, French/snap beans with garlic, carrots and capers. Dried fruit compote.	1 slice date and brazil nut cake.	
(115)	(445)	(160)	1645

Day	Breakfast	Between meal snack	Light meal
Friday	1 glass unsweetened fruit juice Spicy sausages, grilled tomato, wholemeal/ wholewheat toast. (390)	1 slice brunch bread. (140)	Potato omelette. 1 tangerine. (240)
Saturday	1 glass unsweetened fruit juice. Devilled kidneys (360)	1 almond potato cake. (125)	Bean soup, wholemeal/ wholewheat roll. 1 pear. (355)
Sunday	1 glass unsweetened fruit juice. Kedgeree. (275)	1 muesli bar. (175)	Hummus, wholemeal/ wholewheat pitta bread. 1 nectarine. (325)

Between meal snack	Main meal	Between meal snack	Total Kcals
Fruit and nut bites.	Mushroom caps with savoury filling. Sardine bake, ratatouille. Rice dessert.	1 peanut biscuit/ cookie.	
(105)	(340)	(95)	1310
1 cheese scone.	Sweet and sour shallots. Chickpea/garbanzo roast, rosti, vegetable stir- fry. Date and banana pudding.	1 slice All-Bran cake.	
(155)	(450)	(110)	1555
Fruit and nut spread on wholemeal/ wholewheat toast.	Gingery vegetable dip. Chicken with fruit and nuts, pilau rice, beetroot/beet salad. Pineapple kebabs.	1 slice tea bread spread with polyunsaturated margarine.	
(240)	(430)	(200)	1645

About the recipes

All the recipes in this book have been designed to take account of healthy eating guidelines and foods that have been associated with PMS symptoms.

- *Three hourly* portions of complex carbohydrates.
- *Healthy mixture of food* to ensure an adequate supply of essential nutrients.
- *Sugar* in small quantities only. Fresh and dried fruit, and vegetables, such as carrots, have been used as sweetening agents.
- *Complex carbohydrate foods* permeate the recipes, thus ensuring adequate amounts of starch and dietary fibre.
- *Fat* in limited quantities only, and polyunsaturated fat used in preference to saturated fat.
- *Salt* is never added as an actual ingredient, and the use of salty foods in the recipes is minimal.
- *Alcoholic drinks* have not been used.
- *Caffeinated beverages* have not been used.

Key to recipes

Kcals 185	= the number of calories in the specified portion of food is shown here.
½ portion	= The portion size recommended for PMS sufferers
Can be frozen	= The recipe is suitable for freezing at the specified stages. Instructions will need to be obtained from a freezer book.

4

Breakfasts

BRAN MUFFINS

This recipe can also be used as a Between-Meal-Snack.

Serves 6
160 Calories a portion

Metric/Imperial		*American*
115g/4oz	brown flour	1 cup
1 tbs	baking powder/soda	1 tbs
1 tsp	ground cinnamon	1 tsp
55g/2oz	bran	½ cup
1 tbs	soft brown sugar	1 tbs
1	egg, lightly beaten	1
200ml/⅓ pint	semi-skimmed/low fat milk	¾ cup
30g/1oz	melted polyunsaturated margarine	2 tbs

1. Sift (strain) the flour, baking powder (soda) and cinnamon into a large mixing bowl. Tip any remaining bran into the bowl.

2. Add the bran and sugar.
3. Mix the egg, milk and melted fat together in a basin. Then pour the liquid slowly over the flour mixture. Gently fold the mixture together.
4. Spoon the mixture into 12 non-stick or lightly greased bun or muffin tins.
5. Bake in a pre-heated oven set at 400°F/200°C/gas mark 6 for about 20 minutes.
6. Put the muffins on to a cooling rack or serve at once while they are hot. If you wish, spread thinly with polyunsaturated margarine and allow for the extra 40 cals per muffin.

Note to Cooks

Can be frozen.

BREAKFAST COCKTAIL

Serves 1
140 calories a portion

Metric/Imperial		American
1 medium	banana	1 medium
2	stoned/pitted dried dates	2
4 tbs	plain low fat yogurt	4 tbs
1 heaped tbs	wheatgerm	1 heaped tbs

1. Peel and slice the banana.
2. Chop the dates.
3. Put the banana, dates and yogurt into a serving dish and gently fold the mixture together.
4. Sprinkle with the wheatgerm and serve immediately.

BREAKFAST PANCAKES/CRÊPES

Serves 4
235 Calories each

Metric/Imperial		American
4 rashers	lean back bacon	4 slices
1 small	onion	1 small
115g/4oz	wholemeal/wholewheat flour	1 cup
2	eggs	2
140ml/¼ pint	semi-skimmed/low fat milk	⅔ cup
2 tbs	sunflower oil	2 tbs
	freshly milled black pepper	

1. Trim off the bacon rind, gristle and fat and finely chop the lean flesh.
2. Peel and finely dice the onion.
3. Put the bacon and onion into a non-stick pan and fry gently for 5 minutes.
4. Sift (strain) the flour into a large mixing bowl and tip in any remaining bran. Make a well in the centre.
5. Crack the eggs and drop them into the well. Beat the eggs into the flour gradually, taking in the flour from the sides of the bowl.
6. As the mixture begins to thicken add half the milk. When all the flour has been incorporated add the rest of the milk and beat thoroughly.
7. Put the bacon and onion mixture into the batter and mix well.

8. Heat a film of oil in a shallow non-stick frying pan (skillet). Pour in 3 tablespoons of mixture and cook over a moderate heat for 2 minutes. Turn the pancakes (crêpes) over and continue cooking for a further 2 minutes. Put the cooked pancakes (crêpes) on a hot plate and keep warm until the batch is ready.
9. Serve piping hot with a sprinkling of freshly milled black pepper.

Note to Cooks

Can be frozen.

CRUNCHY BREK

Serves 12
240 Calories a portion

Metric/Imperial		American
55g/2oz	soft brown sugar	⅓ cup
140g/5oz	porridge oats	1¼ cups
115g/4oz	chopped hazelnuts	¾ cup
55g/2oz	wheatgerm	½ cup
55g/2oz	sultanas/golden seedless raisins	⅓ cup
1 tbs	sesame seeds	1 tbs
1	orange, zest of	1
140ml/¼ pint	water	⅔ cup
140ml/¼ pint	sunflower oil	⅔ cup

1. Set aside half the sugar. Put the other half into a large mixing bowl with all the dry ingredients.
2. Put the remaining sugar into a basin with the water and oil. Whisk the mixture until it is thoroughly blended.
3. Pour the liquid into the mixing bowl and stir thoroughly.
4. Spread the mixture over a non-stick or lightly oiled baking sheet.
5. Bake in a pre-heated oven set at 375°F/190°C/gas mark 5 for 25 to 30 minutes. During cooking *turn the mixture using a spatula* to ensure it cooks evenly.

6. Leave the mixture on the baking sheet until it has cooled. Store in an airtight container and serve as required. If served with plain low fat yogurt, allow an additional 30 cals and for semi-skimmed/low fat milk 55 cals.

DEVILLED KIDNEYS

Serves 4
295 Calories a portion

Metric/Imperial		American
8	lambs kidneys	8
1 tsp	wholemeal/wholewheat flour	1 tsp
30g/1oz	polyunsaturated margarine	2 tbs
1 tbs	prepared English mustard	1 tbs
1 tbs	mango chutney	1 tbs
1 tsp	wine vinegar	1 tsp
1 tsp	tomato purée/paste	1 tsp
½ tsp	anchovy essence	½ tsp
	Worcestershire sauce	
	cayenne pepper	
4 slices	wholemeal/wholewheat bread	4 slices

1. Prepare the kidneys by cutting them in half and removing their central core and skin. Then cut them into small cubes and toss in the flour.
2. Put the margarine into a shallow non-stick frying pan (skillet) and melt the fat over a low heat. Add the kidneys and fry for 1 minute.
3. Set the kidneys aside. Add the mustard, chutney, vinegar, tomato purée (paste), anchovy essence, dash of Worcestershire sauce and pinch of cayenne pepper to the pan and heat until the sauce is simmering.

4. Add the kidneys and cook for 1 minute over a low heat.
5. Make the toast and pour the devilled kidneys on to it and serve at once.

EGG AND BACON BURGERS

These delicious breakfast burgers can be made the night before, left in the refrigerator and cooked first thing. This recipe can also be used as a Between-Meal-Snack.

Serves 4
230 Calories each

Metric/Imperial		American
225g/½ lb	hot mashed potato	1 cup
1 tbs	beaten egg	1 tbs
2	hard-boiled eggs	2
4 rashers	lean back bacon	4 slices
	Worcestershire sauce	
	freshly milled black pepper	
1	egg, lightly beaten	1
55g/2oz	dried wholemeal/	½ cup
	wholewheat breadcrumbs	
2 tbs	sunflower oil	2 tbs

1. Put the hot mashed potato into a mixing bowl. Add the tablespoon of beaten egg and mix thoroughly.
2. Shell and roughly chop the hard-boiled eggs.
3. Remove any rind, gristle or fat from the bacon. Chop the lean flesh and fry gently in a non-stick pan for 5 minutes.
4. Add the chopped eggs, bacon, dash of Worcestershire sauce and black pepper to the potato mixture and stir well.
5. Shape the mixture into 8 cakes.

6. Coat each cake thoroughly with beaten egg and breadcrumbs.
7. Heat the oil in a shallow non-stick frying pan (skillet) and fry the burgers over a gentle heat until golden brown on each side. Drain on kitchen paper (paper towels).
8. Serve piping hot.

HERRINGS IN APPLE AND OATMEAL

Serves 4
250 Calories a portion

Metric/Imperial		American
4	herring fillets	4
1 medium	eating apple	1 medium
55g/2oz	rolled oats	½ cup
1	egg, lightly beaten	1
1 tbs	sunflower oil	1 tbs

1. Clean the fillets and remove any bones.
2. Peel, core and finely grate the apple.
3. Mix the apple and rolled oats together on a plate.
4. Coat the fish with the beaten egg then press the apple and oat mixture around each fillet.
5. Heat the oil in a shallow non-stick frying pan (skillet) and fry the fillets over a gentle heat for 5 minutes on each side. Drain on kitchen paper (paper towels) and serve hot.

KEDGEREE

As well as a tasty breakfast dish, kedgeree served with green salad makes an appetizing midday or evening meal.

Serves 4
210 Calories a portion

Metric/Imperial		American
225g/½ lb	smoked haddock	½ lb
115g/4oz	brown rice	½ cup
15g/½ oz	polyunsaturated margarine	1 tbs
2 tsps	curry powder	2 tsps
	freshly grated nutmeg	
2 tbs	freshly chopped parsley	2 tbs
2	hard-boiled eggs, sliced	2

1. Poach the haddock, drain and flake and remove any skin or bone.
2. Cook the rice according to the instructions on the packet.
3. Melt the margarine in a large pan over a gentle heat. Add the freshly cooked rice, flaked haddock, curry powder, nutmeg and parsley and toss the mixture, with the lid firmly on the pan, for 30 seconds.
4. Pile the kedgeree loosely in a hot serving dish and garnish with the slices of egg.

Note to Cooks

Can be frozen at stage 3.

MUESLI

Serves 1
370 Calories a portion

Metric/Imperial		American
1 tbs	oat flakes	1 tbs
1 tbs	rye flakes	1 tbs
1 tbs	chopped hazelnuts	1 tbs
1 tbs	sultanas/golden seedless raisins	1 tbs
4 tbs	plain low fat yogurt	4 tbs
1	apple, grated	1
1 tbs	fresh orange juice	1 tbs
1 tbs	wheatgerm	1 tbs

1. Put the oat flakes and rye flakes into a basin. Cover them with water and soak overnight. Drain thoroughly before use.
2. Place the prepared flakes, nuts, sultanas (golden seedless raisins), yogurt, apple and orange juice in a bowl. Mix the ingredients together thoroughly.
3. Sprinkle with wheatgerm just before serving.

SPICY SAUSAGES

These spicy sausages can be prepared the night before, stored in a refrigerator and cooked first thing. Alternatively they may be frozen for future use. This recipe can also be used as a Between-Meal-Snack.

Serves 4
230 Calories each

Metric/Imperial		American
455g/1 lb	lean minced pork	1 lb
55g/2oz	fresh wholemeal/ wholewheat breadcrumbs	1 cup
1 tbs	freshly chopped sage	1 tbs
1 tsp	dried mace	1 tsp
	freshly milled black pepper	
1 tbs	water	1 tbs
1 tbs	sunflower oil	1 tbs

1. Put the pork, breadcrumbs, flavourings and water into a mixing bowl and stir thoroughly, using a fork.
2. Form the mixture into 8 sausage shapes.
3. Heat the oil in a shallow non-stick frying pan (skillet) and fry the sausages over a moderate heat for 15 minutes. Reduce the temperature as necessary and turn the sausages to ensure even cooking.
4. Drain the sausages on kitchen paper (paper towels).
5. Serve hot. This dish goes well with grilled tomatoes (20 cals) and wholemeal (wholewheat) toast (75 cals).

Note to Cooks
Can be frozen at stages 2 or 4.

Between-meal-snacks

ALMOND POTATO CAKES

Serves 12
125 Calories each

Metric/Imperial		American
340g/¾ lb	mashed potato	1½ cups
	freshly grated nutmeg	
1 tbs	wholemeal/wholewheat flour	1 tbs
1	egg, lightly beaten	1
140g/5oz	chopped almonds	1 cup
2 tbs	sunflower oil	2 tbs

1. Flavour the mashed potato with the freshly grated nutmeg.
2. Shape the potato into 12 rounds.
3. Coat with flour, then brush with the beaten egg. Press the chopped almonds on to the surface of the cakes.
4. Heat half the oil in a shallow non-stick frying pan (skillet). Cook 6 of the cakes over a moderate heat for

3 minutes. Turn the cakes over and continue cooking for 3 more minutes. Cook the remaining 6 cakes in the same way, using the reserved oil.

5. Drain on kitchen paper (paper towels).
6. Chill and use as required.

Note to Cooks

Can be frozen at stages 3 or 5.

BAKED BEAN BURGERS

Serves 8
140 Calories each

Metric/Imperial		American
1 x 450g	can baked beans	2 cups
140g/5oz	fresh wholemeal/ wholewheat breadcrumbs	2½ cups
4tbs	cooked, diced lean bacon	4 tbs
	Worcestershire sauce	
	freshly milled black pepper	
1	egg, lightly beaten	1
30g/1oz	dried wholemeal/ wholewheat breadcrumbs	¼ cup
2 tbs	sunflower oil	2 tbs

1. Pour the baked beans into a sieve (strainer) over a basin and leave for 15 minutes to let the sauce drain away. Stir the beans periodically to speed the process up.
2. Put the drained beans into a large mixing bowl and mash thoroughly.
3. Add the fresh breadcrumbs, bacon and flavourings and stir well.
4. Shape the mixture into 12 rounds and coat with the egg and dried breadcrumbs.
5. Heat 1 tablespoon of oil in a large shallow non-stick frying pan (skillet) and fry 6 of the burgers for 3 minutes on each side. Drain on kitchen paper (paper towels). Repeat the process with the remaining burgers.

6. Chill and serve as required.

Note to Cooks

Can be frozen.

CHEESE SCONES

Serves 8
155 Calories each

Metric/Imperial		American
200g/7oz	self-raising wholemeal/ self-rising wholewheat flour	1¾ cups
1 tsp	mustard powder	1 tsp
30g/1oz	polyunsaturated margarine	2 tbs
85g/3oz	Cheddar/hard cheese, grated	¾ cup
120ml/4 fl oz	semi-skimmed/low fat milk	¼ cup

1. Sift (strain) the flour and mustard powder into a large mixing bowl. Tip any remaining bran into the bowl.
2. Add the margarine and rub this into the flour using the tips of the fingers until the flour mixture resembles fine breadcrumbs.
3. Add two-thirds of the cheese and stir well.
4. Gradually add the milk so that the mixture is soft but not wet.
5. Lightly knead the dough on a floured work surface until the mixture looks smooth. Roll out to 1.8cm (¾ in) thickness and cut into rounds using a 5cm (2 in) cutter. Leave for 15 minutes, then brush with milk and sprinkle with the remaining cheese.
6. Heat a baking sheet and put the scones on to it, and without delay, bake in a pre-heated oven set at 450°F/230°C/gas mark 8 for 8 to 10 minutes.

7. Cool the scones on a rack.
8. Pack in an airtight container and keep up to 3 days.

Note to Cooks

Can be frozen.

CRAB BITES

Serves 4
150 Calories each

Metric/Imperial		American
170g/6oz	canned crabmeat	1 cup
85g/3oz	fresh wholemeal/ wholewheat breadcrumbs	1½ cups
2 tbs	freshly chopped parsley	2 tbs
1 tsp	creamed horseradish	1 tsp
½ tsp	freshly squeezed lemon juice	½ tsp
1	egg, separated	1
30g/1oz	dried wholemeal/ wholewheat breadcrumbs	¼ cup
1 tbs	sunflower oil	1 tbs

1. Put the crab, fresh breadcrumbs, parsley, horse-radish, lemon juice and egg yolk into a large mixing bowl. Stir the mixture thoroughly to blend the ingredients together.
2. Divide the mixture into 8 and shape into rounds.
3. Coat with the egg white and dried breadcrumbs.
4. Heat the oil in a large shallow non-stick frying pan (skillet). Fry the rounds for 3 minutes over a moderate heat then turn them over and continue cooking for 3 more minutes. Drain thoroughly on kitchen paper (paper towels).
5. Chill and use as required.

Note to Cooks

Can be frozen at stages 3 or 4.

GARLIC BITES

Serves 4
110 Calories a portion

Metric/Imperial		American
4 cloves	garlic	4 cloves
1 tbs	sunflower oil	1 tbs
4 slices	wholemeal/wholewheat bread	4 slices

1. Peel and crush (mince) the garlic.
2. Pour the oil on to a baking sheet and add the garlic. Stir the mixture well and spread evenly on the baking sheet.
3. Trim the crusts off the bread (these can be used to make breadcrumbs) and cut the bread into 1cm (½ in) cubes.
4. Tip the cubes of bread on to the baking sheet and turn them over so that the surfaces are coated with the oil mixture.
5. Bake in a pre-heated oven set at 350°F/180°C/gas mark 4 for 8 to 10 minutes.
6. When thoroughly cool store in an airtight container until required.

POTATO AND PARSNIP CAKES

Serves 12
120 Calories each

Metric/Imperial		American
170g/6oz	mashed potato	¾ cup
170g/6oz	mashed parsnip	¾ cup
115g/4oz	chopped cashew nuts	¾ cup
	freshly grated nutmeg	
1 tbs	wholemeal/wholewheat flour	1 tbs
1	egg, lightly beaten	1
55g/2oz	dried wholemeal/wholewheat breadcrumbs	½ cup
2 tbs	sunflower oil	2 tbs

1. Put the mashed potato and parsnip into a large mixing bowl. Add the chopped nuts and nutmeg and stir thoroughly.
2. Shape the mixture into 12 rounds.
3. Coat with the flour, then brush with the beaten egg. Finally coat with the breadcrumbs.
4. Heat half the oil in a shallow non-stick frying pan (skillet). Cook 6 cakes over a moderate heat for 3 minutes. Turn the cakes over and continue cooking for a further 3 minutes.
5. Drain the cakes on kitchen paper (paper towels). Cook the other cakes in the same way using the remaining oil.

6. Chill and use as required.

Note to Cooks

Can be frozen at stages 3 or 5.

POTATO AND SPINACH CAKES

Serves 12
115 Calories each

Metric/Imperial		American
1 small	onion	1 small
2 cloves	garlic	2 cloves
1 tsp	sunflower oil	1 tsp
225g/½ lb	frozen spinach, de-frosted	1 cup
455g/1 lb	mashed potato	2 cups
115g/4oz	grated Cheddar/ hard cheese	1 cup
	freshly milled black pepper	
1 tbs	wholemeal/wholewheat flour	1 tbs
1	egg, lightly beaten	1
55g/2oz	dried wholemeal/ wholewheat breadcrumbs	½ cup
1 tbs	sunflower oil	1 tbs

1. Peel and grate the onion.
2. Peel and crush (mince) the garlic.
3. Heat the teaspoon of oil in a shallow non-stick frying pan (skillet). Add the onion and garlic and fry over a low heat to soften the onion mixture.
4. Thoroughly drain the spinach and add this to the onion mixture with the potato, cheese and freshly milled black pepper. Stir thoroughly.
5. Shape the mixture into 12 rounds.
6. Coat with the flour then brush with the beaten egg. Finally coat with the breadcrumbs.

Between-meal-snacks

7. Heat half the oil in a large shallow non-stick frying pan (skillet). Cook 6 of the cakes over a moderate heat for 3 minutes. Turn the cakes over and continue cooking for a further 3 minutes.
8. Drain on kitchen paper (paper towels). Cook the other cakes in the same way using the remaining oil.
9. Chill and use as required.

Note to Cooks

Can be frozen at stages 5 or 8.

BEAN DIP

Serves 4
215 Calories a portion

Metric/Imperial		American
1 small	onion	1 small
2 cloves	garlic	2 cloves
225g/½ lb	cooked or canned flageolet beans	1⅓ cups
1 tbs	freshly squeezed lemon juice	1 tbs
1 tbs	sunflower oil	1 tbs
2 tbs	tomato purée/paste	2 tbs
2 tbs	freshly chopped coriander/cilantro	2 tbs
4	wholemeal/wholewheat pitta breads (to serve)	4

1. Peel and chop the onion.
2. Peel and crush (mince) the garlic.
3. Put the onion, garlic, drained beans, lemon juice, sunflower oil, tomato purée (paste) and coriander (cilantro) into the goblet of a food processor and process to form a smooth paste.
4. Chill in a covered container and take portions as required. Serve with wholemeal (wholewheat) pitta bread.

PEANUT DIP

Serves 8
205 Calories a portion

Metric/Imperial		American
2 medium	bananas	2 medium
2	spring onions/scallions	2
225g/½ lb	chopped roasted peanuts	1½ cups
1 small	lemon, juice and zest	1 small
1 tbs	tomato purée/paste	1 tbs
140ml/¼ pint	plain low fat yogurt	⅔ cup
55g/2oz	fresh wholemeal/ wholewheat breadcrumbs	1 cup
16 sticks	celery (to serve)	16 stalks

1. Peel and roughly chop the bananas.
2. Trim, wash and chop the spring onions (scallions).
3. Put the bananas, spring onions (scallions), peanuts, juice and zest of the lemon, tomato purée (paste) and yogurt into the goblet of a liquidizer/blender or food processor and process to form a paste.
4. Tip the mixture into a mixing bowl and add the breadcrumbs. Stir thoroughly.
5. Chill in a covered container and take portions as required. Serve with sticks (stalks) of celery.

PASTA SALAD WITH TUNA

Serves 1
200 Calories a portion

Metric/Imperial		American
½ portion	pasta salad (p. 164)	½ portion
30g/1oz	tuna, flaked	2 tbs

1. Mix the pasta salad and tuna together in a small basin.
2. Pile the mixture into a small container with a lid, and chill.

POTATO SALAD WITH HAM

Serves 1
125 Calories a portion

Metric/Imperial		American
½ portion	potato salad (p. 160)	½ portion
30g/1oz	diced lean ham	2 tbs

1. Mix the potato salad and ham together in a small basin.
2. Pile the mixture into a small container with a lid, and chill.

TABBOULEH WITH PEANUTS

Serves 1
200 Calories a portion

Metric/Imperial		American
½ portion	tabbouleh (p. 166)	½ portion
15g/½oz	roasted peanut kernels	1 tbs

1. Mix the tabbouleh and peanuts together in a small basin.
2. Pile the mixture into a small container with a lid, and chill.

VEGETABLE RICE WITH CHICKEN

Serves 1
170 Calories a portion

Metric/Imperial		American
½ portion	vegetable rice (p. 167)	½ portion
30g/1oz	cooked diced chicken	2 tbs

1. Mix the vegetable rice and chicken together in a small basin.
2. Pile the mixture into a small container with a lid, and chill.

CASHEW AND LENTIL LOAF

10 slices
145 Calories a slice

Metric/Imperial		*American*
1 small	onion	1 small
115g/4oz	mushrooms	2 cups
1 tsp	sunflower oil	1 tsp
170g/6oz	green lentils	1 cup
425ml/¾ pint	vegetable stock	2 cups
115g/4oz	chopped cashew nuts	¾ cup
55g/2oz	fresh wholemeal/ wholewheat breadcrumbs	1 cup
2 tbs	freshly chopped marjoram	2 tbs
1 tbs	soya/soy sauce	1 tbs
1	egg, lightly beaten	1

1. Peel and finely dice the onion.
2. Wipe and finely chop the mushrooms.
3. Heat the oil in a heavy based casserole or saucepan. Add the onion and fry over a low heat until softened.
4. Add the mushrooms, lentils and stock. Put the lid on the pan and simmer for 1 hour. Stir periodically. Towards the end of cooking remove the lid from the pan and let the moisture evaporate.
5. Stir in the cashew nuts, breadcrumbs, marjoram, soya (soy) sauce and egg.
6. Spoon the mixture into a non-stick or lightly greased and lined 455g (1 lb) loaf tin. Cover the surface with foil.

7. Bake in a pre-heated oven set at 375°F/190°C/gas mark 5 for about 50 minutes.
8. Let the loaf settle in the tin for 10 minutes then turn it on to a flat plate. Cut into slices when cold.

Note to Cooks

Can be frozen.

CHEESY LOAF

12 slices
150 Calories a slice

Metric/Imperial		American
55g/2oz	Bran-Buds	1¼ cups
140ml/¼ pint	semi-skimmed/low fat milk	⅔ cup
225g/½ lb	self-raising/rising brown flour	2 cups
	cayenne pepper	
55g/2oz	polyunsaturated margarine	¼ cup
115g/4oz	grated Cheddar/ hard cheese	1 cup
2 sticks	celery, finely diced	2 stalks
1	egg, lightly beaten	1

1. Put the Bran-Buds in a basin and add the milk. Stir well and leave the mixture to stand for 30 minutes.
2. Sift (strain) the flour with a pinch of cayenne pepper into a large mixing bowl. Tip any remaining bran into the bowl.
3. Add the margarine to the flour and rub the mixture together using the tips of the fingers.
4. When it resembles breadcrumbs add the cheese, celery, Bran-Buds and egg. Stir well.
5. Place the mixture in a non-stick or lightly greased and lined 455g (1 lb) loaf tin.
6. Bake in a pre-heated oven set at 375°F/190°C/gas mark 5 for about 50 minutes.

7. Leave the loaf to stand for 15 minutes and then turn it on to a cooling rack.

8. When cool, wrap in aluminium foil and keep for up to 5 days.

Note to Cooks

Can be frozen.

STILTON LOAF

12 slices
195 Calories a slice

Metric/Imperial		American
225g/½ lb	self-raising/rising brown flour	2 cups
½ tsp	baking powder/soda	½ tsp
55g/2oz	polyunsaturated margarine	¼ cup
115g/4oz	crumbled Stilton/blue veined cheese	1 cup
115g/4oz	chopped walnuts/English walnuts	¾ cup
1	egg, lightly beaten	1
140ml/¼ pint	semi-skimmed/low fat milk	⅔ cup

1. Sift (strain) the flour and baking powder (soda) into a large mixing bowl. Tip any remaining bran into the bowl.
2. Add the margarine and rub the fat into the flour until the mixture resembles breadcrumbs.
3. Add the cheese and walnuts and stir well.
4. Mix the egg and milk together and add the liquid to the dry ingredients.
5. Pour the mixture into a non-stick or lightly greased and lined 455g (1 lb) loaf tin.
6. Bake in a pre-heated oven set at 375°F/190°C/gas mark 5 for about 1 hour.
7. Leave the loaf to stand in the tin for 15 minutes then put it on to a cooling rack.

8. When cool wrap in aluminium foil and keep for up to 5 days.

Note to Cooks

Can be frozen.

FRUIT AND NUT BITES

Serves 4
160 Calories a portion

Metric/Imperial		American
55g/2oz	chopped dried dates	⅓ cup
55g/2oz	chopped dried apricots	⅓ cup
55g/2oz	chopped dried figs	⅓ cup
55g/2oz	chopped hazelnuts	½ cup
30g/1oz	fresh wholemeal/ wholewheat breadcrumbs	½ cup
1 tbs	freshly squeezed orange juice	1 tbs

1. Mince the dried fruits using a hand mincer or food processor.
2. Put the mixture into a large mixing bowl.
3. Add half the chopped nuts and all the fresh breadcrumbs and orange juice and mix thoroughly using a fork.
4. Shape the mixture into 12 2.5cm (1 in) rounds.
5. Coat with the remaining finely chopped nuts.
6. Chill thoroughly and keep in an airtight container in a refrigerator. Use within 3 days.

MUESLI BARS

Makes 12
175 Calories each

Metric/Imperial		American
55g/2oz	seedless raisins	⅓ cup
60ml/2 fl oz	unsweetened orange juice	¼ cup
90ml/3 fl oz	sunflower oil	⅓ cup
55g/2oz	finely chopped apple	⅓ cup
85g/3oz	chopped dried apricots	½ cup
115g/4oz	wholemeal/wholewheat flour	1 cup
30g/1oz	low fat soya flour	¼ cup
115g/4oz	porridge oats	1 cup

1. Put the raisins and orange juice in the goblet of a liquidizer (blender) or food processor and process for 30 seconds.
2. Pour the liquid into a mixing bowl and add the oil, apple and dried apricots.
3. Add the flours and porridge oats and stir the mixture thoroughly.
4. Spread the mixture in a non-stick or lightly greased baking tray 30x20cm (12x8in) and bake for 30 minutes in a pre-heated oven set at 350°F/180°C/gas mark 4.
5. Leave the mixture in the tin and mark into 12 slices while still warm.
6. When thoroughly cooled store in an airtight container. Keep for up to 1 week.

OATY BISCUITS/COOKIES

Makes 24
65 Calories each

Metric/Imperial		American
140g/5oz	wholemeal/wholewheat flour	1¼ cups
1 tsp	baking powder/soda	1 tsp
115g/4oz	polyunsaturated margarine	½ cup
55g/2oz	medium oatmeal	½ cup
15g/½ oz	soft brown sugar	1 tbs
1 tbs	semi-skimmed/low fat milk	1 tbs

1. Sift (strain) the flour and baking powder (soda) into a large mixing bowl. Tip any remaining bran into the bowl.
2. Cut the fat up in the flour and rub the mixture together using the tips of the fingers. Continue rubbing in until the mixture looks like fine breadcrumbs.
3. Add the oatmeal, sugar and milk and stir until the mixture holds together.
4. Roll the mixture out thinly on a lightly floured work surface. Cut into rounds using a 5cm (2 in) cutter. Lightly pierce the surface of the biscuits (cookies) with a fork.
5. Bake on two lightly greased or non-stick baking sheets in a pre-heated oven set at 350°F/180°C/gas mark 4 for 15 minutes or until browned.

6. Leave the biscuits (cookies) on the baking sheets for 10 minutes; then carefully transfer them on to a cooling rack.
7. When thoroughly cooled store in an air-tight container. Keep up to 1 week.

BRUNCH BREAD

18 slices
140 Calories a slice

Metric/Imperial		American
55g/2oz	Bran-Buds	1¼ cups
140ml/¼ pint	semi-skimmed/low fat milk	⅔ cup
115g/4oz	polyunsaturated margarine	½ cup
115g/4oz	soft brown sugar	⅔ cup
2	eggs, lightly beaten	2
170g/6oz	dried apricots (no soak variety)	1 cup
55g/2oz	chopped hazelnuts	½ cup
115g/4oz	self-raising/rising brown flour	1 cup

1. Put the Bran-Buds in a basin and add the milk. Leave the mixture to stand for 30 minutes.
2. Cream the fat and sugar together in a large mixing bowl. Gradually beat in the eggs.
3. Stir in the fruit and nuts and soaked Bran-Buds.
4. Gently fold in the flour.
5. Pour the mixture into a non-stick or lightly greased and lined 900g (2 lb) loaf tin.
6. Bake in a pre-heated oven set at 350°F/180°C/gas mark 4 for 1 to 1¼ hours.
7. Leave the cake to stand for 15 minutes and then turn it on to a cooling rack.
8. When thoroughly cooled wrap in aluminium foil and keep up to 1 week.

Between-meal-snacks

Note to Cooks

Can be frozen.

CARROT AND HAZELNUT CAKE

This is my favourite cake. It improves with keeping and is beautifully moist.

12 slices
120 Calories a slice

Metric/Imperial		American
3 size 1	eggs	3 large
115g/4oz	brown sugar	⅔ cup
170g/6oz	grated carrot	1 cup
140g/5oz	chopped hazelnuts	1 cup
1 medium	lemon, zest of	1 medium
55g/2oz	wholemeal/wholewheat flour	½ cup
½ tsp	baking powder/soda	½ tsp

1. Separate the egg whites from the yolks.
2. Whisk the yolks with the sugar in a large mixing bowl until the mixture is thick and creamy.
3. Add the grated carrot, hazelnuts and lemon zest and fold the mixture together.
4. Sift (strain) the flour and baking powder (soda) into the mixture. Tip any remaining bran into the bowl. Gently fold the mixture together.
5. Whisk the egg whites into stiff peaks and fold them into the ingredients in the mixing bowl.
6. Pour the cake mixture into a non-stick or lightly greased and lined 18cm (7 in) square cake tin.
7. Bake in a pre-heated oven set at 350°F/180°C/gas mark 4 for about 40 minutes.

Between-meal-snacks

8. Leave the cake to stand for 15 minutes, then turn it on to a cooling rack.
9. When cold wrap in aluminium foil and keep up to 1 week.

FRUIT AND NUT SPREAD

Serves 12
240 Calories a portion

Metric/Imperial		American
85g/3oz	chopped dried figs	½ cup
85g/3oz	chopped dried dates	½ cup
85g/3oz	stoned/pitted raisins	½ cup
225g/½ lb	coarsely chopped hazelnuts	1⅔ cups
55g/2oz	fresh wholemeal/ wholewheat breadcrumbs	1 cup
55g/2oz	fromage frais	¼ cup
½	lemon zest	½
4 tbs	fresh orange juice	4 tbs
1 tbs	sunflower oil	1 tbs
12 slices	wholemeal/wholewheat toast (to serve)	12 slices

1. Put all the ingredients, except the toast, into the goblet of a food processor and blend.
2. Spoon the spread into a container with a lid and store in the refrigerator for up to 1 week.
3. Serve as required with slices of hot wholemeal (wholewheat) toast.

Note to Cooks

Can be frozen.

TEA BREAD

12 slices
160 Calories a slice

Metric/Imperial		American
55g/2oz	sultanas/golden seedless raisins	⅓ cup
55g/2oz	chopped dates	⅓ cup
55g/2oz	chopped figs	⅓ cup
55g/2oz	seedless raisins	⅓ cup
55g/2oz	mixed peel	⅓ cup
1	orange, zest of	1
1 tsp	mixed spice	1 tsp
140ml/¼ pint	herbal tea	⅔ cup
225g/½ lb	self-raising/rising brown flour	2 cups
2 tsp	baking powder/soda	2 tsp
2	eggs, lightly beaten	2
4 tbs	sunflower oil	4 tbs

1. Put the fruit, orange zest, mixed spice and herbal tea into a large bowl. Stir the mixture thoroughly and leave for about 8 hours.

2. Sift (strain) the flour and baking powder (soda) into a large mixing bowl. Tip any remaining bran into the bowl.

3. Add the fruit mixture, eggs and oil and mix thoroughly.

4. Pour the mixture into a non-stick or lightly greased and lined 455g (1 lb) loaf tin.

5. Bake in a pre-heated oven set at 350°F/180°C/gas mark 4 for 40 minutes, then reduce the temperature to 325°F/170°C/gas mark 3.

6. Leave the tea bread in the tin for 15 minutes and then put on to a cooling rack.

7. This can be served with a very thin spread of polyunsaturated margarine, but will add about 40 cals.

8. To store tea bread wrap in aluminium foil and keep for up to 5 days.

Note to Cooks

Can be frozen.

Light meals

JACKET POTATOES

Serves 1
120 Calories each

Metric/Imperial		*American*
1 medium	potato	1 medium

Fillings

Bacon and sweetcorn   *115 Calories a portion*

55g/2oz	cooked diced bacon	⅓ cup
30g/1oz	cooked sweetcorn kernels	2 tbs
1 tsp	French mustard	1 tsp

Cheese and mango chutney   *150 Calories a portion*

30g/1oz	Cheddar/hard cheese, grated	¼ cup
1 tbs	mango chutney	1 tbs

Chicken, yogurt and mint   85 Calories a portion

55g/2oz	cooked diced chicken	⅓ cup
1 tbs	plain low fat yogurt	1 tbs
1 tbs	fresh chopped mint	1 tbs

Sausage, apple and sage   180 Calories a portion

55g/2oz	cooked pork sausage, sliced	⅓ cup
1 tbs	apple purée	1 tbs
1 tsp	freshly chopped sage	1 tsp

Tuna and mayonnaise   200 Calories a portion

55g/2oz	canned tuna, flaked	⅓ cup
1 tbs	low calorie mayonnaise	1 tbs
1 tbs	freshly chopped parsley	1 tbs

1. Scrub and score the potato all around with the point of a sharp knife.
2. To achieve a crunchy skin, bake the potato for about 1 hour or until soft in a pre-heated oven set at 400°F/200°C/gas mark 6. Otherwise, cook in a microwave oven following the model's instructions.
3. Cut the potato in half and scoop out the flesh. Leave the skin intact.
4. Mash the flesh in a mixing bowl and mix with the chosen filling.
5. Pile the mixture into the potato skin and finish cooking. Allow 10 minutes in a conventional oven, or time specified by microwave cooking instructions.

PITTA POCKETS

This recipe can be used as a Between-Meal-Snack.

Serves 1
120 Calories a portion

Metric/Imperial		American
1 medium	wholemeal/wholewheat pitta bread	1 medium

Fillings

Egg, mustard and cress and mayonnaise
120 Calories per portion

1	hard-boiled egg, chopped	1
15g/½ oz	mustard and cress	½ cup
1 tbs	low calorie mayonnaise	1 tbs

Feta cheese, tomato and onion   150 Calories a portion

55g/2oz	feta cheese, cubed	½ cup
1 medium	tomato, sliced	1 medium
2	spring onions/scallions, chopped	2

Smoked tofu, lettuce and watercress
45 Calories a portion

55g/2oz	smoked tofu, cubed	⅓ cup
2 leaves	cos/romaine lettuce, shredded	2 leaves
15g/½ oz	watercress	½ cup

Tuna, cucumber and yogurt   *170 Calories a portion*

55g/2oz	canned tuna, flaked	⅓ cup
10 slices	cucumber	10 slices
1 tbs	plain low fat yogurt	1 tbs

1. Mix the ingredients for the selected filling in a small basin.
2. Slit the pitta open with a sharp knife and pack the filling inside.

RÖSTI MEALS

Serves 1
160 Calories a portion

Metric/Imperial		American
1 medium	waxy potato	1 medium
	freshly milled black pepper	
1 tsp	polyunsaturated margarine	1 tsp

Toppings

Bacon and tomato   *100 Calories a portion*

55g/2oz	lean bacon, cooked and diced	⅓ cup
1 small	tomato, grilled and chopped	1 small

Poached egg and parsley   *80 Calories a portion*

1	poached egg	1
1 tbs	freshly chopped parsley	1 tbs

Sausage and beans   *215 Calories a portion*

55g/2oz	grilled sausage, diced	⅓ cup
2 tbs	baked beans, cooked	2 tbs

Smoked tofu and mushroom   *45 Calories a portion*

55g/2oz	smoked tofu, cooked	⅓ cup
1 tbs	mushrooms, sliced and stewed	1 tbs

Swiss cheese   225 Calories a portion

2 slices   Gruyère cheese   2 slices

1. Parboil the potato in its skin for approximately 10 minutes. Allow to cool.
2. Peel the potato and grate on to a work surface or plate. Sprinkle with freshly milled black pepper and gently fold the mixture together.
3. Heat ½ teaspoon margarine in a small non-stick shallow frying pan (skillet).
4. Add the potato and flatten using a round-bladed knife. Cook over a moderate heat for 10 minutes.
5. Put a flat plate over the top of the pan and invert the pan so that the potato falls neatly on to the plate.
6. Put the remaining margarine into the pan. When it has melted slide the potato mixture back into the pan. Cook for a further 10 minutes.
7. Slip the rösti on to a hot plate and arrange the chosen topping on the surface.

CHEESE AND MUSHROOM PÂTÉ

Serves 4
170 Calories a portion

Metric/Imperial		American
170g/6oz	mushrooms	3 cups
1 small	onion	1 small
15g/½ oz	polyunsaturated margarine	1 tbs
30g/1oz	fresh wholemeal/ wholewheat breadcrumbs	½ cup
170g/6oz	cottage/pot cheese	¾ cup
2 tbs	freshly chopped parsley	2 tbs
1 small	lemon, zest of freshly grated nutmeg	1 small
4 slices	wholemeal/wholewheat toast (to serve)	4 slices

1. Wipe and roughly chop the mushrooms.
2. Peel and slice the onion.
3. Melt the margarine in a shallow non-stick frying pan (skillet). Add the onion and fry over a low heat for 5 minutes.
4. Add the mushrooms and continue cooking with the lid on the pan for 10 more minutes.
5. Pour the mixture into the goblet of a liquidizer (blender) or a food processor and add the breadcrumbs, cottage (pot) cheese, parsley, lemon zest and nutmeg. Process until smooth.
6. Arrange the mixture in a pâté dish and chill.

7. Serve with hot slices of wholemeal (wholewheat) toast.

Note to Cooks

Can be frozen.

CHEESY PUDDING

Serves 4
160 Calories a portion

Metric/Imperial		American
285ml/½ pint	semi-skimmed/low fat milk	1⅓ cups
55g/2oz	fresh brown breadcrumbs	1 cup
2	eggs	2
1 tsp	dried mustard powder	1 tsp
	freshly milled black pepper	
55g/2oz	Cheddar/hard cheese, grated	½ cup
1 tsp	sunflower oil	1 tsp

1. Heat the milk in a non-stick saucepan. Add the bread-crumbs, put the lid on the pan and leave the mixture to cool for 30 minutes.
2. Separate the egg yolks and whites.
3. Add the egg yolks, mustard powder, pepper and cheese to the milk and bread mixture. Stir thoroughly.
4. Whisk the egg whites until stiff peaks have formed and fold into the cheese mixture.
5. Lightly oil a 285ml (1 pt) ovenproof dish. Pour the mixture into the dish and bake in a pre-heated oven set at 350°F/180°C/gas mark 4.
6. Bake for 30 minutes or until the pudding is golden brown and well risen.
7. Serve at once. This dish goes well with vegetables or a mixed salad.

GLAMORGAN SAUSAGES

This recipe can also be used as a Between-Meal-Snack.

Serves 6
190 Calories each

Metric/Imperial		American
115g/4oz	mature Cheddar/hard cheese, grated	1 cup
140g/5oz	fresh wholemeal/ wholewheat breadcrumbs	2½ cups
1 small	onion	1 small
1 tsp	dried mixed herbs	1 tsp
1 tsp	dried mustard powder	1 tsp
	freshly milled black pepper	
2	eggs, lightly beaten	2
30g/1oz	dried wholemeal/ wholewheat breadcrumbs	¼ cup
1 tbs	sunflower oil	1 tbs

1. Put the cheese and fresh breadcrumbs into a mixing bowl.
2. Peel and grate the onion and add this to the cheese and breadcrumbs.
3. Add the mixed herbs, mustard and pepper.
4. Add half the beaten egg to the cheese mixture and stir well. When the mixture holds together, divide it into 12 sausage shapes.
5. Dip the sausages into the remaining beaten egg and coat with the dried breadcrumbs.

6. Heat the oil in a shallow non-stick frying pan (skillet). Fry the sausages over a medium heat for 5 minutes. Turn to ensure even cooking.
7. Drain the sausages on kitchen paper (paper towels).
8. Serve hot or cold. This dish goes well with mixed salad.

Note to Cooks

Can be frozen at stages 5 or 7.

POTATO PIZZA

This recipe can also be used as a Between-Meal-Snack.

Serves 6
275 Calories a portion

Metric/Imperial		*American*
Base		
225g/½ lb	potatoes	½ lb
55g/2oz	polyunsaturated margarine	¼ cup
115g/4oz	self-raising wholemeal/ self-rising wholewheat flour	1 cup
	freshly grated nutmeg	
Topping		
1 large	onion	1 large
115g/4oz	mushrooms	2 cups
1 large	red/sweet pepper	1 large
1 clove	garlic	1 clove
2 tsps	sunflower oil	2 tsps
1 tbs	freshly chopped oregano or marjoram	1 tbs
3 tbs	tomato purée/paste	3 tbs
115g/4oz	mature Cheddar/hard cheese, grated	1 cup

1. Scrub, peel, boil and mash the potatoes.
2. Add the margarine, flour and nutmeg and mix to form a dough.

3. Roll the dough to form a 25cm (10 in) round and place on a non-stick or lightly greased baking sheet.
4. Peel and dice the onion.
5. Wipe and thinly slice the mushrooms.
6. De-seed, wash and finely dice the pepper.
7. Peel and crush (mince) the garlic.
8. Heat the oil in a shallow non-stick frying pan (skillet). Add the onion and garlic and fry gently for 5 minutes. Add the mushrooms, pepper and fresh herb and fry for one more minute.
9. Spread the tomato purée (paste) over the pizza base. Spread the vegetable mixture over the top and cover with the cheese.
10. Bake in a pre-heated oven set at 400°F/200°C/gas mark 6 for 30 minutes.
11. Serve hot or cold. This dish goes well with a salad of tomatoes and basil.

Note to Cooks

Can be frozen.

POTATO OMELETTE - PERSIAN STYLE

This is an adventurous way of using up left-over mashed potato.

Serves 1
215 Calories a portion

Metric/Imperial		American
55g/2oz	mashed potato	¼ cup
1	egg	1
2	spring onions/scallions	2
	freshly milled black pepper	
2 tsps	sunflower oil	2 tsps

1. Put the potato into a mixing bowl.
2. Beat the egg in a basin and add this to the potato. Stir thoroughly.
3. Chop the spring onions (scallions) and add these with the pepper to the potato and egg paste. Stir well.
4. Heat 1 teaspoon oil in a shallow non-stick frying pan (skillet). Spread the mixture evenly in the pan and cook over a low heat for 5 minutes.
5. Place a flat plate over the top of the pan; invert the pan so that the omelette falls neatly on to the plate. Put the rest of the oil into the pan and slide the omelette into it. Cook for 5 more minutes.
6. Serve hot.

SCRAMBLES ON TOAST

This savoury scramble is a delicious breakfast treat.

Serves 1
270 Calories a portion

Metric/Imperial		American
1 slice	wholemeal/wholewheat bread	1 slice
1	egg	1
1 tbs	semi-skimmed/low fat milk freshly milled black pepper	1 tbs
15g/½oz	sunflower margarine	1 tbs

Variations

Bacon   95 Calories a portion

55g/2oz	diced, cooked lean bacon	⅓ cup

Cheese   125 Calories a portion

30g/1oz	Cheddar/hard cheese, grated	¼ cup

Mushroom and marjoram   7 Calories a portion

55g/2oz	finely chopped mushrooms	¼ cup
1 tsp	finely chopped marjoram	1 tsp

Smoked haddock and parsley   55 Calories a portion

55g/2oz	smoked haddock, cooked and flaked	⅓ cup
1 tbs	freshly chopped parsley	1 tbs

1. Make the toast and keep it warm.
2. Crack the egg into a small basin.
3. Add the milk and black pepper and beat well.
4. Heat the margarine in a non-stick saucepan. Add the egg mixture and your favourite variation. Stir continuously over a moderate heat until the egg mixture is set.
5. Pile the scramble on to the hot toast and serve without delay.

KIPPER PÂTÉ

This recipe can also be used as a Between-Meal-Snack.

Serves 6
165 Calories a portion

Metric/Imperial		American
225g/½ lb	kipper fillets	½ lb
4 tbs	plain low fat yogurt	4 tbs
1 tbs	horseradish cream	1 tbs
1 tbs	lemon juice	1 tbs
55g/2oz	mashed potato	¼ cup
	freshly milled black pepper	
6 slices	wholemeal/wholewheat bread (to serve)	6 slices

1. Cook the kipper fillets and allow to cool.
2. Put all the ingredients into the goblet of a food processor or a liquidizer (blender) and process to a purée.
3. Pour the mixture into a pâté dish and chill for 30 minutes.
4. Serve as a spread with slices of wholemeal (wholewheat) toast.

Note to Cooks

Can be frozen.

SALMON FISHCAKES

You can make these using tuna or any cooked fish. The recipe can also be used as a Between-Meal-Snack.

Serves 4
260 Calories each

Metric/Imperial		*American*
225g/½ lb	mashed potato	1 cup
225g/½ lb	salmon, canned	1⅓ cups
30g/1oz	freshly chopped parsley	1 cup
1 small	lemon, zest of	1 small
1 tsp	anchovy essence	1 tsp
2	eggs, lightly beaten	2
1 tbs	wholemeal/wholewheat flour	1 tbs
55g/2oz	dried wholemeal/ wholewheat breadcrumbs	½ cup
1 tbs	sunflower oil	1 tbs

1. Put the cold mashed potato into a mixing bowl.
2. Drain the salmon and flake it, using a fork. Add salmon to the potato.
3. Add the parsley, lemon zest, anchovy essence and half the egg and fold the mixture together.
4. Sprinkle the flour on a work surface and roll the fish mixture into a sausage shape. Cut into 8 cakes and shape into rounds.
5. Dip each cake in the remaining egg and ensure every crevice is covered. Then coat with the dried bread-crumbs.

6. Heat the oil in a shallow non-stick frying pan (skillet). Cook the fishcakes over a moderate heat for 3 minutes on each side. Drain thoroughly on kitchen paper (paper towels).

7. Serve hot with a selection of freshly cooked vegetables or cold with salad.

Note to Cooks

Can be frozen at stages 5 or 6.

BEEFBURGERS

Serves 4
205 Calories each

Metric/Imperial		American
1 small	onion	1 small
225g/½ lb	lean ground beef	½ lb
	freshly milled black pepper	
½ tsp	dried mixed herbs	½ tsp
½ tsp	mushroom ketchup/	½ tsp
	catsup	
4	soft wholemeal/wholewheat	4
	baps/buns (to serve)	

1. Peel and grate the onion.
2. Put the onion, beef, pepper, herbs and ketchup (catsup) into a mixing bowl and mix thoroughly.
3. Shape the mixture into 4 even size burgers about 1cm (½ in) thick. A hamburger press is a convenient way of ensuring an even shape.
4. Pre-heat a grill (broiler) and cook the beefburgers under a moderate heat for 3 minutes on each side.
5. Lightly toast the baps/buns and serve the beefburgers inside them.

Note to Cooks

Can be frozen at stages 3 or 4.

SCOTCH EGGS

This recipe can also be used as a Between-Meal-Snack.

Serves 4
245 Calories each

Metric/Imperial		American
4	eggs	4
225g/½ lb	low fat sausage meat	½ lb
1 tsp	dry mustard powder	1 tsp
½ tsp	dried sage	½ tsp
1 tbs	wholemeal/wholewheat flour	1 tbs
1	egg, lightly beaten	1
55g/2oz	dried wholemeal/ wholewheat breadcrumbs	½ cup

1. Hard-boil the eggs, cool thoroughly and remove the shells.
2. Mix the sausage meat with the mustard and dried sage. Shape into 4 even-size round cakes.
3. Dust the eggs with the flour and wrap a portion of sausage meat around each egg. Press out any cracks and be sure to keep the sausage to an even thickness.
4. Dip the sausage meat coated eggs in beaten egg and coat thoroughly with the dried breadcrumbs.
5. Bake the eggs on a non-stick baking sheet in a pre-heated oven set at 400°F/200°C/gas mark 6 for 20 minutes.
6. Serve hot or cold with a variety of salads.

BEAN SOUP

Serves 4
310 Calories a portion

Metric/Imperial		American
115g/4oz	haricot/navy beans	½ cup
1 large	onion	1 large
1 large	carrot	1 large
1 stick	celery	1 stalk
2 cloves	garlic, crushed/minced	2 cloves
1 tbs	sunflower oil	1 tbs
2 tbs	tomato purée/paste	2 tbs
1	bouquet garni	1
570ml/1 pint	water	2½ cups
1 tsp	yeast extract	1 tsp
1 tbs	freshly chopped marjoram	1 tbs
285ml/½ pint	skimmed/low fat milk	1⅓ cups
4	crusty wholemeal/ wholewheat rolls (to serve)	4

1. Soak the beans for about 8 hours or overnight and drain well.
2. Peel and chop the onion and carrot. Scrub and chop the celery.
3. Heat the oil in a large heavy pan, add the prepared vegetables and garlic and fry over a gentle heat for 3 minutes to lightly brown them.
4. Add the tomato purée (paste), bouquet garni, beans and water and bring the mixture to boiling point and boil for 15 minutes. Put the lid on the pan and simmer for 2 hours.

Light meals

5. Use a liquidizer (blender) or food processor to process the mixture to form a purée. Pour the purée into a clean pan.
6. Add the yeast extract and freshly chopped marjoram and milk and cook over a gentle heat for 5 minutes.
7. Serve steaming hot in a soup tureen with the wholemeal (wholewheat) bread rolls.

Note to Cooks

Can be frozen.

FALAFEL

This recipe can also be used as a Between-Meal-Snack.

Serves 4
130 Calories a portion

Metric/Imperial		American
285g/10oz	chickpeas/garbanzos, cooked or canned	1½ cups
1 clove	garlic, crushed/minced	1 clove
55g/2oz	fresh wholemeal/ wholewheat breadcrumbs	1 cup
30g/1oz	freshly chopped parsley	1 cup
½ tsp	ground coriander/cilantro	½ tsp
½ tsp	ground cumin	½ tsp
1 tbs	sunflower oil	1 tbs

1. Thoroughly drain the chickpeas (garbanzos).
2. Put the chickpeas (garbanzos), garlic, breadcrumbs, parsley and spices into the goblet of a liquidizer (blender) or food processor and process to a smooth paste.
3. Using the palms of the hands, form the mixture into 2.5cm (1 in) balls.
4. Heat the oil in a shallow non-stick frying pan (skillet). Fry the balls over a moderate heat for about 5 minutes. Shake the pan (skillet) periodically to ensure even cooking.
5. Drain the falafel on kitchen paper (paper towels).

6. Serve hot or cold. This tasty savoury dish goes well with salads and yogurt.

Note to Cooks

Can be frozen at stages 3 or 5.

SPICY LENTIL SOUP

Serves 4
225 Calories a portion

Metric/Imperial		American
170g/6oz	red lentils	1 cup
850ml/1½ pints	water	3¾ cups
½ tsp	ground turmeric	½ tsp
2	green chillies	2
2 cloves	garlic	2 cloves
1 tsp	sunflower oil	1 tsp
½ tsp	mustard seeds	½ tsp
1 tbs	desiccated coconut	1 tbs
170g/6oz	cooked brown rice	1 cup
1 tbs	freshly chopped coriander/ cilantro	1 tbs

1. Put the lentils into a heavy based pan. Add the water and turmeric and bring the mixture to boiling point. Simmer with the lid on the pan for 20 minutes or until thoroughly cooked.
2. De-seed the chillies, rinse and dice finely.
3. Peel and crush (mince) the garlic.
4. Heat the oil in a small pan. Add the chillies, garlic and mustard seeds. Fry over a moderate heat until the mustard seeds have popped.
5. Add the coconut and continue cooking for 2 minutes.
6. When the lentils are cooked, add the spicy mixture and cooked rice and continue cooking for 5 more minutes.

Light meals

7. Serve in a hot soup tureen sprinkled with the coriander (cilantro).

Note to Cooks

Can be frozen.

HUMMUS

This recipe can be used as a Between-Meal-Snack.

Serves 6
275 Calories a portion

Metric/Imperial		American
285g/10oz	chickpeas/garbanzos, cooked or canned	1½ cups
2 cloves	garlic	2 cloves
85g/3oz	tahini	⅓ cup
1 tbs	lemon juice	1 tbs
1 tbs	sunflower oil	1 tbs
60ml/2 fl oz	water	¼ cup
	cayenne pepper	
1 tbs	freshly chopped parsley	1 tbs
6 medium	wholemeal/wholewheat pitta breads (to serve)	6 medium

1. Thoroughly drain the chickpeas (garbanzos).
2. Peel and crush (mince) the garlic.
3. Put the chickpeas (garbanzos), garlic, tahini, lemon juice, sunflower oil, water and pinch of cayenne pepper into the goblet of a liquidizer (blender) or food processor and process to a smooth mixture that resembles mayonnaise.
4. Pour the mixture into a serving dish and sprinkle with the parsley.
5. Serve chilled with wholemeal (wholewheat) pitta bread.

Light meals

LENTIL BURGERS

This recipe can be used as a Between-Meal-Snack.

Serves 4
250 Calories a portion

Metric/Imperial		American
115g/4oz	red lentils	½ cup
55g/2oz	mushrooms	1 cup
2 sticks	celery	2 stalks
170g/6oz	carrot, grated	1 cup
1 tbs	freshly chopped marjoram or oregano	1 tbs
55g/2oz	fresh wholemeal/ wholewheat breadcrumbs	1 cup
2	eggs, lightly beaten	2
1 tbs	wholemeal/wholewheat flour	1 tbs
55g/2oz	dried wholemeal/ wholewheat breadcrumbs	½ cup
1 tbs	sunflower oil	1tbs

1. Boil the lentils in 570ml (1 pt) or 2½ cups of water for 20 to 25 minutes. Drain well.
2. Wipe and very finely chop the mushrooms.
3. Scrub, string and very finely chop the celery.
4. Put the lentils, mushrooms, celery, carrot, marjoram or oregano, fresh breadcrumbs and half the egg into a mixing bowl and stir thoroughly.

5. Shape the mixture into a sausage shape on a floured work surface. Cut into 8 rounds and coat with the remaining flour.
6. Dip each burger in the remaining beaten egg and coat thoroughly with the breadcrumbs.
7. Heat the oil in a shallow non-stick frying pan (skillet). Cook the burgers for 5 minutes on each side. Drain on kitchen paper (paper towels).
8. Serve hot with fresh vegetables or cold with salad.

Note to Cooks

Can be frozen at stages 6 or 7.

MINTY LENTIL SALAD

This recipe can also be used as a Between-Meal-Snack.

Serves 6
295 Calories a portion

Metric/Imperial		American
225g/½ lb	brown lentils	1 cup
8	spring onions/scallions	8
1 small	lemon, juice of	1 small
2 tbs	sunflower oil	2 tbs
2 tbs	freshly chopped mint	2 tbs
4	lemon wedges	4
4	crusty wholemeal/ wholewheat rolls (to serve)	4

1. Pour the lentils into a large pan and cover them with water. Bring to boiling point and simmer for 30 minutes. Drain thoroughly.
2. Trim, wash and dice the spring onions (scallions).
3. Put the freshly cooked hot lentils into a large bowl. Add the spring onions (scallions), lemon juice, sunflower oil and mint. Toss the mixture thoroughly so that the lentils absorb all the flavours.
4. Leave to cool. Serve chilled garnished with the wedges of lemon and crusty wholemeal (wholewheat) rolls.

7

Main meals

STARTERS

AVOCADO WITH FRUIT

Serves 4
90 Calories ½ portion

Metric/Imperial		American
1 large	orange	1 large
1 medium	grapefruit	1 medium
24	seedless white grapes	24
1 medium	ripe avocado pear	1 medium
1 tbs	olive oil	1 tbs
1 tsp	lemon juice	1 tsp
	freshly milled black pepper	
	dry mustard powder	
4 sprigs	fresh mint	4 sprigs

1. Peel and segment the orange and grapefruit. Remove the pips. Wash and dry the grapes.

2. Peel, stone (pit) the avocado pear and cut into thin slices.
3. Shake the olive oil, lemon juice, pepper and pinch of mustard in a small jar.
4. Arrange the avocado slices and fruit in 4 individual dishes and sprinkle with the dressing.
5. Chill for 15 minutes and serve with sprigs of fresh mint.

GAZPACHO

A delicious soup to serve on very hot days. Add two to three ice cubes to each serving to make it even more refreshing.

Serves 4
50 Calories ½ portion

Metric/Imperial		American
455g/1 lb	tomatoes	1 lb
1 medium	green/bell pepper	1 medium
2 cloves	garlic	2 cloves
55g/2oz	fresh wholemeal/ wholewheat breadcrumbs	1 cup
2 tbs	white wine vinegar	2 tbs
1 tbs	olive oil	1 tbs
2 tbs	iced water	2 tbs

Garnish

½ small	cucumber	½ small
1 small	tomato	1 small
1 small	green/bell pepper	1 small

1. Remove the skins from the tomatoes and de-seed.
2. Wash, de-seed and roughly chop the green (bell) pepper.
3. Peel and crush (mince) the garlic.
4. Put the tomatoes, pepper, garlic, breadcrumbs, vinegar and oil into the goblet of a liquidizer (blender) or food processor and process until smooth.

5. Add the iced water and pour the mixture into a large bowl. Cover and chill in the refrigerator for at least 1 hour.
6. Prepare the garnish. Peel and finely dice the cucumber; skin, de-seed and finely dice the tomato; and wash, de-seed and finely dice the green(bell) pepper.
7. Serve the soup in individual soup bowls sprinkled with the garnish.

LENTIL PÂTÉ

A delicious filling for lunch time sandwiches. This recipe can also be used as a Between-Meal-Snack.

Serves 6
120 Calories ½ portion

Metric/Imperial		American
225g/½ lb	red lentils	1 cup
225g/½ lb	potatoes	½ lb
1 large	onion	1 large
1 large	carrot	1 large
3 cloves	garlic, crushed/minced	3 cloves
2 tbs	freshly chopped thyme	2 tbs
1 tsp	sunflower oil	1 tsp
6 slices	wholemeal/wholewheat toast (to serve)	6 slices

1. Pour the lentils into a large heavy based pan and cover with water. Boil for 20 minutes. Drain any remaining liquid.
2. Peel and chop the potatoes, onion and carrot. Rinse under cold running water and cook the vegetables in enough boiling water to just cover them. Boil until tender and drain well.
3. Put the lentils, vegetables, garlic and thyme into the goblet of a food processor and blend to form a purée.
4. Pour the mixture into an ovenproof dish and brush the surface lightly with sunflower oil.

5. Bake in an oven pre-heated to 400°F/200°C/gas mark 6 for 20 minutes.
6. Allow to cool and serve chilled with wholemeal (wholewheat) toast.

Note to Cooks

Can be frozen.

LENTIL SOUP

Lentil soup served with chunky wholemeal (whole-wheat) bread makes a nutritious light meal in its own right.

Serves 4
100 Calories ½ portion

Metric/Imperial		American
225g/½ lb	red lentils	1 cup
850ml/1½ pints	vegetable stock	3¾ cups
1 large	onion	1 large
2 cloves	garlic	2 cloves
1 tsp	sunflower oil	1 tsp
½ tsp	ground coriander/cilantro	½ tsp
½ tsp	ground cumin	½ tsp
4 wedges	lemon	4 wedges

1. Pour the lentils into a large heavy based pan, add the stock and bring the mixture to boiling point.
2. Simmer for 30 minutes and remove any scum that rises to the surface, using a slotted spoon.
3. Peel and chop the onion.
4. Peel and crush (mince) the garlic.
5. Heat the oil in a non-stick frying pan (skillet) over a moderate heat. Fry the onion and garlic until brown. Add the coriander (cilantro) and continue cooking for 1 minute.
6. Add the ground cumin to the lentils and stir well.

7. Serve the soup in individual bowls garnished with the onion mixture and a wedge of lemon.

Note to Cooks

Can be frozen at stage 2.

MUSHROOM PÂTÉ

This recipe can also be used as a Between-Meal-Snack.

Serves 4
95 Calories ½ portion

Metric/Imperial		American
1 small	onion	1 small
1 clove	garlic	1 clove
1 tsp	sunflower oil	1 tsp
225g/½ lb	mushrooms, chopped	3 cups
30g/1oz	fresh wholemeal/ wholewheat breadcrumbs	½ cup
1	egg, beaten	1
1 tsp	tomato purée/paste	1 tsp
2 tbs	freshly chopped marjoram	2 tbs
	freshly milled black pepper	
4	wholemeal/wholewheat bread rolls (to serve)	4

1. Peel and finely dice the onion.
2. Peel and crush (mince) the garlic.
3. Heat the oil in a non-stick frying pan (skillet) and fry the onion and garlic over a gentle heat to soften them.
4. Add the mushrooms and continue cooking for a further 5 minutes.
5. Add the breadcrumbs and stir over the heat for about 2 minutes. Using a beating action add the egg.
6. Add the tomato purée (paste), herbs and freshly milled black pepper. Stir thoroughly.

7. Pour the mixture into a pâté dish and chill for 1 hour before serving.
8. Serve with crusty wholemeal (wholewheat) bread rolls.

Note to Cooks

Can be frozen.

MUSHROOM CAPS
WITH SAVOURY FILLING

This flavoursome dish can also be served as a light meal.

Serves 4
105 Calories ½ portion

Metric/Imperial		American
4 large	field mushrooms	4 large
4 rashers	lean back bacon	4 slices
1 small	onion	1 small
1 tbs	sunflower oil	1 tbs
55g/2oz	fresh wholemeal/ wholewheat breadcrumbs	1 cup
1 tsp	freshly chopped thyme	1 tsp
1 tbs	freshly chopped parsley	1 tbs
1	lemon, zest of	1
1	egg, lightly beaten	1
1 tbs	grated Parmesan cheese	1 tbs
4 slices	wholemeal/wholewheat bread	4 slices

1. Wipe the mushrooms and remove the stalks. Keep the cups intact but finely chop the stalks.
2. Remove any rind and fat from the bacon and dice the lean flesh.
3. Peel and finely dice the onion.
4. Glaze a non-stick shallow frying pan (skillet) with a film of sunflower oil and heat gently.

5. Add the bacon, onion and chopped mushroom stalks. Cook for 5 minutes.

6. Add the breadcrumbs, herbs and lemon zest. Stir thoroughly. Remove from the heat and stir in the egg.

7. Pile the mixture into the mushroom caps and sprinkle them with the Parmesan cheese. Arrange the filled mushrooms in a lightly oiled ovenproof dish and brush the mushrooms with any remaining oil.

8. Bake in an oven set at 400°F/200°C/gas mark 6 for 20 to 25 minutes.

9. Cut the bread into 6.25cm (2½ in) rounds using a pastry cutter, and toast under a pre-heated grill (broiler).

10. Serve the mushrooms on the croûtons.

TANGY CARROT SOUP

Serves 4
20 Calories ½ portion

Metric/Imperial		American
455g/1 lb	carrots	1 lb
1 small	onion	1 small
1 tsp	sunflower oil	1 tsp
850ml/1½ pints	vegetable stock	3¾ cups
1	orange, zest and juice	1
1 tbs	freshly chopped coriander/ cilantro	1 tbs
½ tsp	paprika	½ tsp

1. Peel or scrape, rinse and chop the carrots.
2. Peel and chop the onion.
3. Heat the oil in a heavy based pan. Add the onion and fry over a gentle heat for 5 minutes.
4. Add the carrots and continue cooking for 2 minutes.
5. Add the stock, zest and juice of the orange, coriander (cilantro) and paprika. Bring the mixture to boiling point and leave to simmer with the lid on the pan for 45 minutes.
6. Pour the soup into the goblet of a liquidizer (blender) or food processor and process until it is smooth.
7. Rinse the pan. Return the soup to the pan and heat until piping hot.
8. Serve with garlic croûtons (garlic bites p. 58); a half portion will yield an extra 55 cals.

Note to Cooks
Can be frozen.

POTATO DIP

This recipe can also be used as a Between-Meal-Snack.

Serves 4
70 Calories ½ portion

Metric/Imperial		American
225g/½ lb	potatoes	½ lb
1 large	onion	1 large
1 tsp	sunflower oil	1 tsp
2 tsps	caraway seeds	2 tsps
225g/½ lb	cottage cheese/pot cheese	1 cup
	freshly milled black pepper	
8 sticks	celery (to serve)	8 stalks
8	baby carrots (to serve)	8

1. Peel and cube the potatoes. Peel and slice the onion.
2. Cook the vegetables in enough boiling water to just cover them. Boil the vegetables until tender and drain thoroughly.
3. Put the vegetables into a large mixing bowl and mash them.
4. Heat the oil in a pan and add the caraway seeds. Cook over a gentle heat for 1 minute and stir continuously.
5. Pass the cottage (pot) cheese through a sieve (strainer).
6. Mix the mashed vegetables, caraway seeds, cheese and pepper.
7. Serve chilled with the sticks (stalks) of celery and the baby carrots.

GINGERY VEGETABLE DIP

This recipe can also be used as a Between-Meal-Snack.

Serves 4
50 Calories ½ portion

Metric/Imperial		American
455g/1 lb	young carrots	1 lb
225g/½ lb	swede/rutabaga	½ lb
225g/½ lb	potatoes	½ lb
1 large	orange, zest and juice	1 large
1 tbs	freshly chopped ginger root	1 tbs
2 tbs	plain low fat yogurt	2 tbs

1. Scrape the carrots, cut half into chunks and the rest into fingers. Set the fingers aside.
2. Peel and slice the swede (rutabaga).
3. Peel and slice the potatoes.
4. Cook the prepared vegetables in enough boiling water to just cover them until tender. Drain thoroughly.
5. Put the cooked vegetables into the goblet of a liquidizer (blender) or food processor and process to a purée. Leave to cool.
6. Put the orange zest and juice into the goblet of the liquidizer (blender) or food processor with the ginger and yogurt and blend together.
7. Mix all the ingredients (except the carrot fingers) together.
8. Serve chilled with the carrot fingers.

SWEET AND SOUR SHALLOTS

Serves 4
25 Calories ½ portion

Metric/Imperial		American
20	shallots	20
1 tbs	olive oil	1 tbs
1 tbs	white wine vinegar	1 tbs
1 tsp	brown sugar	1 tsp
2 tbs	freshly chopped parsley	2 tbs

1. Peel the shallots.
2. Heat the oil in a shallow non-stick frying pan (skillet) and fry the shallots over a gentle heat for 10 minutes. Shake the pan to ensure even cooking.
3. Add the vinegar, sugar and just enough water to cover the shallots. Simmer with the lid off the pan for 1 hour.
4. Leave the mixture to cool and pour into 4 individual dishes. Chill for 30 minutes and sprinkle with the parsley.

MAIN DISHES

CHEESE AND VEGETABLE BAKE

This recipe can also be used as a Between-Meal-Snack.

Serves 6
90 Calories ½ portion

Metric/Imperial		American
170g/6oz	mushrooms	3 cups
1 small	onion	1 small
1 large	green/bell pepper	1 large
1 stick	celery	1 stalk
1 tbs	sunflower oil	1 tbs
170g/6oz	fresh wholemeal/ wholewheat breadcrumbs	3 cups
115g/4oz	Cheddar/hard cheese, grated	1 cup
1	egg, lightly beaten	1
1 tbs	freshly chopped sage	1 tbs

1. Wipe and chop the mushrooms finely.
2. Peel and finely dice the onion.
3. Wash, de-seed and dice the pepper very finely.
4. Scrub and finely dice the celery.
5. Heat the oil in a shallow non-stick frying pan (skillet). Add the onion and fry over a low heat for 5 minutes.
6. Add the mushrooms, pepper and celery and continue cooking for a further 5 minutes.
7. Turn the heat source off and add the breadcrumbs, cheese, egg and sage. Mix thoroughly.

8. Pour the mixture into a non-stick, or lightly greased and lined 455g (1 lb) loaf tin and spread evenly.

9. Bake in a pre-heated oven set at 375°F/190°C/gas mark 5 for 1 hour and 10 minutes.

10. Leave the mixture to stand in the tin for 15 minutes to settle.

11. Serve hot. This dish goes well with jacket potato and mixed salad or a selection of fresh vegetables and tomato sauce.

Note to Cooks

Can be frozen.

PESTO

Any pesto that is left may be spread on fresh wholemeal (wholewheat) bread and used as a Between-Meal-Snack or light meal.

Serves 6
150 Calories ½ portion

Metric/Imperial		*American*
55g/2oz	fresh basil leaves	2 cups
2 tbs	toasted pine nuts	2 tbs
3 cloves	garlic, crushed/minced	3 cloves
90ml/3 fl oz	sunflower oil	⅓ cup
55g/2oz	Parmesan cheese, grated	½ cup
455g/1 lb	fresh wholemeal/ wholewheat pasta	1 lb

1. Put the basil, pine nuts, garlic and oil into the goblet of a liquidizer (blender) or food processor and process to a smooth paste.
2. Pour the mixture into a basin and stir in the cheese.
3. Cook the pasta according to the packet instructions. Drain thoroughly.
4. Serve the pesto with the piping hot pasta and freshly grated Parmesan cheese. This dish goes well with mixed side salad and crusty wholemeal (wholewheat) bread rolls to mop up the delicious sauce.

EGG CURRY

Serves 4
100 Calories ½ portion

Metric/Imperial		American
1 medium	onion	1 medium
1 large clove	garlic	1 large clove
1 tbs	sunflower oil	1 tbs
1 medium	carrot	1 medium
3 sticks	celery	3 stalks
1 medium	eating apple	1 medium
2 tsps	curry powder	2 tsps
½ tsp	turmeric	½ tsp
1 large	tomato	1 large
200ml/⅓ pint	water	¾ cup
200ml/⅓ pint	plain low fat yogurt	¾ cup
6	eggs	6

1. Peel and slice the onion and crush (mince) the garlic.
2. Heat the oil in a heavy based pan and add the onion and garlic. Fry over a low heat for 5 minutes.
3. Peel and dice the carrot and celery; core, peel and dice the apple. Add the prepared vegetable and fruit mixture to the pan with the curry powder and turmeric. Fry over a low heat for 5 minutes.
4. Skin, de-seed and chop the tomato and add to the pan with the water. Bring the mixture to simmering point; put the lid on the pan and simmer for 20 minutes.
5. Hard-boil the eggs, shell them and set aside.

6. Pour the curry mixture into the goblet of a liquidizer (blender) or food processor and process until smooth.
7. Pour the sauce into a clean pan and add the yogurt. Cook for 3 to 5 minutes.
8. Cut the eggs in half lengthways and arrange them in a shallow dish with the rounded sides facing upwards. Cover with the sauce and serve hot. This dish goes well with pilau rice (see p. 165).

EGG AND SPINACH CAKE

This recipe can also be used as a Between-Meal-Snack.

Serves 8
105 Calories ½ portion

Metric/Imperial		American
225g/½ lb	frozen spinach	1 cup
225g/½ lb	risotto rice	1 cup
1 medium	onion	1 medium
1 tsp	sunflower oil	1 tsp
3	eggs	3
115g/4oz	freshly grated Parmesan cheese	1 cup
	freshly milled black pepper	
	freshly grated nutmeg	

1. Defrost, drain and chop the spinach.
2. Cook the rice according to the instructions on the packet.
3. Peel and finely dice the onion.
4. Put the oil in a shallow non-stick frying pan (skillet), add the onion and fry over a moderate heat until the onion is light brown.
5. Put the spinach, rice and onion into a large bowl.
6. Crack the eggs and lightly beat the whites and yolks together.
7. Add the eggs, cheese, pepper and nutmeg to the spinach, rice and onion mixture. Stir thoroughly.

8. Spread the mixture evenly in a lightly oiled ring mould or cake tin.

9. Bake in a pre-heated oven set at 400°F/200°C/gas mark 6 for 30 minutes.

10. Serve hot. This dish goes well with mixed side salad.

Note to Cooks

Can be frozen.

FISH PIE

Metric/Imperial		American
455g/1 lb	smoked haddock	1 lb
2	eggs	2
30g/1oz	polyunsaturated margarine	2 tbs
30g/1oz	wholemeal/wholewheat flour	¼ cup
140ml/¼ pint	fish stock	⅔ cup
140ml/¼ pint	semi-skimmed/low fat milk	⅔ cup
115g/4oz	shelled prawns/shrimps	1 cup
2 tbs	freshly chopped parsley	2 tbs
	freshly grated nutmeg	
455g/1lb	mashed potato	2 cups
30g/1oz	mature Cheddar/hard cheese, grated	¼ cup

1. Poach the haddock in a shallow pan for 10 minutes. Remove any scum that rises to the surface. Retain the cooking liquor for stock.
2. Remove any skin and bones and flake the fish, using a fork.
3. Hard-boil the eggs, cool and shell them, then chop.
4. Heat the margarine in a non-stick saucepan. Add the flour and stir, using a wooden spoon, to form a roux. This should take about 1 minute.

5. Remove the pan from the heat; gradually stir in the fish stock, beating the mixture smooth with a wooden spoon. Stir in the milk.

6. Return the pan to the heat, bring the sauce to boiling point and stir vigorously to prevent any lumps from forming. Cook the sauce for 3 minutes until it is thickened and smooth.

7. Add the prawns (shrimps), parsley, flaked haddock and chopped eggs and lightly fold the mixture together.

8. Tip the mixture into a shallow ovenproof dish and spread evenly.

9. Stir the freshly grated nutmeg into the mashed potato and spread the potato over the fish mixture. Smooth the surface with a knife. Mark the surface using a fork to make a pattern.

10. Bake in a pre-heated oven set at 425°F/220°C/gas mark 7 for 30 minutes. Sprinkle the cheese on the surface and continue cooking for a further 10 minutes.

11. Serve piping hot. This dish goes well with any green vegetable.

Note to Cooks

Can be frozen at stages 8 or 9.

POTATO TOPPED WITH MACKEREL

Serves 4
125 Calories ½ portion

Metric/Imperial		American
455g/1 lb	potatoes	1 pound
2 tbs	sunflower oil	2 tbs
2 cloves	garlic, crushed/minced	2 cloves
4 tbs	freshly chopped parsley	4 tbs
	freshly milled black pepper	
4	mackerel fillets	4

1. Peel and slice the potatoes very thinly.
2. Mix the oil, garlic, parsley and pepper together in a small basin.
3. Pour half the oil mixture into an ovenproof dish. Add the potatoes and stir thoroughly.
4. Bake in a pre-heated oven set at 450°F/230°C/gas mark 8 for 15 minutes.
5. Take the dish out of the oven. Arrange the mackerel fillets on top of the potato and sprinkle with the remaining oil mixture. Put the dish back in the oven and continue cooking for a further 15 minutes.
6. Serve hot. This dish goes well with mixed salad.

Note to Cooks

Can be frozen.

SARDINE BAKE — ITALIAN STYLE

Serves 4
130 Calories ½ portion

Metric/Imperial		American
680g/1½ lbs	fresh sardines	1½ lbs
455g/1 lb	potatoes	1 lb
1 tbs	sunflower oil	1 tbs
2 cloves	garlic	2 cloves
4 tbs	freshly chopped parsley	4 tbs
115g/4oz	tomatoes, skinned, de-seeded and chopped	⅔ cup
1 tsp	freshly chopped oregano or marjoram	1 tsp
	freshly milled black pepper	

1. Clean and bone the sardines.
2. Scrub, peel and cut the potatoes into 1cm (½ in) slices.
3. Put most of the oil into a shallow frying pan (skillet) and heat. Add the potatoes and fry over a moderate heat for 5 minutes.
4. Lightly oil the base of a 30cm (12 in) baking tin with the remaining oil.
5. Crush (mince) the garlic and spread this in the oil. Sprinkle with the parsley and arrange the potatoes, overlapping as necessary, on the base of the tin.
6. Put the fish on top then cover with the tomatoes.
7. Sprinkle with oregano or marjoram and pepper.
8. Bake in a pre-heated oven set at 350°F/180°C/gas mark 4 for 30 minutes.

Main meals

9. Serve hot. This dish goes well with a mixed side salad.

Note to Cooks

Can be frozen.

CHILLI CON CARNE

This dish is ideally made the day before it is required to allow the flavours to develop. Chill in the refrigerator until needed and re-heat thoroughly.

Serves 4
125 Calories ½ portion

Metric/Imperial		American
455g/1 lb	lean stewing steak	1 lb
1 tsp	sunflower oil	1 tsp
170g/6oz	onion, chopped	1 cup
1 large clove	garlic, crushed/minced	1 large clove
1 medium	green/bell pepper	1 medium
1 tsp	chilli powder	1 tsp
2 tbs	tomato purée/paste	2 tbs
455g/1 lb	canned chopped tomatoes	2¼ cups
285g/10oz	red kidney beans, cooked or canned	1½ cups

1. Remove any fat from the meat. Cut the meat into cubes and then mince.
2. Heat the oil in a deep non-stick pan/casserole. Add the meat and brown over a moderate heat. Set the meat aside.
3. Add the onion and garlic to the pan and fry over a low heat for 5 minutes. Meanwhile, de-seed, core and dice the pepper. Add this to the pan and cook for 2 more minutes.

4. Add the chilli powder, tomato purée (paste), chopped tomatoes and meat. Stir well and bring the mixture to simmering point.
5. Put the lid on the pan and cook for about 1 hour.
6. Drain the red kidney beans and add these to the mixture and cook for 5 more minutes.
7. Serve steaming hot. This tasty dish goes very well with jacket potatoes or crusty garlic bread, green side salad and chilled plain low fat yogurt.

Note to Cooks

Can be frozen at stage 5.

LAMB WITH DRIED FRUIT

Serves 4
185 Calories ½ portion

Metric/Imperial		American
1 medium	aubergine/eggplant	1 medium
1 large	onion	1 large
1 tsp	sunflower oil	1 tsp
455g/1 lb	lean lamb, cubed	1 lb
½ tsp	cinnamon	½ tsp
¼ tsp	allspice	¼ tsp
70g/2½oz	dried dates, stoned/pitted	½ cup
70g/2½oz	dried apricots	½ cup
55g/2oz	blanched almonds	½ cup

1. Trim, wash and cut the aubergine (eggplant) into cubes. Spread the aubergine (eggplant) on a plate and sprinkle with salt. Leave for about 30 minutes and rinse thoroughly under cold running water to remove the bitter juices and salt.
2. Peel and slice the onion.
3. Heat the oil in a heavy based casserole and add the onion. Fry gently to soften the onion.
4. Add the meat and continue cooking for 5 minutes or until the meat is brown all over.
5. Add enough water to just cover the meat and onion. Sprinkle with the cinnamon and allspice. Bring the mixture to boiling point. Put the lid on the pan and simmer for 1 hour.

6. Add the aubergine (eggplant) and dried fruit and continue cooking for 30 minutes.
7. Toast the almonds under a moderately hot grill (broiler).
8. Serve hot sprinkled with the toasted almonds. This dish goes well with pilau rice (see p. 165).

Note to Cooks

Can be frozen.

TOAD-IN-THE-HOLE

Serves 4
200 Calories ½ portion

Metric/Imperial		American
115g/4oz	brown flour	1 cup
2	eggs, lightly beaten	2
285ml/½ pint	semi-skimmed/low fat milk	1⅓ cups
1 tbs	sunflower oil	1 tbs
455g/1 lb	low fat pork sausages	1 lb

1. Sift (strain) the flour into a mixing bowl. Tip into the bowl any remaining bran.
2. Make a well in the flour by pushing it to the sides of the bowl using the back of a wooden spoon.
3. Drop the eggs into the well and add half the milk. Beat the liquid so that the flour gradually falls into it. Beat until a smooth cream has formed.
4. Stir in the rest of the milk.
5. Put the oil and sausages into a non-stick baking tin about 20x25cm (8x10 in) and place in a pre-heated oven set at 425°F/220C/gas mark 7. Cook for 5 minutes.
6. Pour the batter into the tin, over the sausages, and return the tin to the hot oven.
7. Bake for 45 minutes until the batter is well risen and brown.
8. Serve without delay. This dish goes well with fresh vegetables and onion gravy.

CHICKEN WITH FRUIT AND NUTS

Serves 4
195 Calories ½ portion

Metric/Imperial		American
4	chicken portions on the bone	4
1 medium	onion	1 medium
115g/4oz	blanched almonds	1 cup
115g/4oz	sultanas/golden seedless raisins	⅔ cup
115g/4oz	chopped dried apricots	⅔ cup
185ml/⅓ pint	chicken stock	1⅓ cup
½ tsp	ground ginger	½ tsp
½ tsp	ground cinnamon	½ tsp
¼ tsp	turmeric	¼ tsp
4 tbs	freshly chopped parsley	4 tbs

1. Remove the skin and underlying fat from the chicken portions.
2. Peel and slice the onion.
3. Put the chicken, onion, almonds, sultanas (golden seedless raisins), chopped apricots, stock and spices into a heavy based pan.
4. Bring the mixture to boiling point, then cover and simmer over a gentle heat for 45 minutes.
5. Add the parsley and continue cooking for a further 5 minutes.
6. Serve piping hot with brown rice or jacket potato and side salad.

CHICKEN AND TARRAGON SALAD

Serves 4
120 Calories ½ portion

Metric/Imperial		*American*
340g/¾ lb	cooked white chicken	2⅓ cups
140ml/¼ pint	low calorie mayonnaise	⅔ cup
140ml/¼ pint	plain low fat yogurt	⅔ cup
2 tbs	freshly chopped tarragon	2 tbs

1. Remove any skin from the chicken and cut the meat into strips.
2. Mix the mayonnaise, yogurt and tarragon together in a large basin and gently fold in the chicken.
3. Chill and serve with a variety of salads.

CHICKPEA/GARBANZO ROAST

This recipe can also be used as a Between-Meal-Snack.

Serves 4
95 Calories ½ portion

Metric/Imperial		American
1 tbs	sunflower oil	1 tbs
170g/6oz	onion, finely diced	1 cup
2 cloves	garlic, crushed, minced	2 cloves
2 tbs	tomato purée/paste	2 tbs
1 tbs	freshly chopped oregano or marjoram	1 tbs
	freshly milled black pepper	
340g/¾ lb	chickpeas/garbanzos, canned or cooked	1⅓ cups
115g/4oz	fresh wholemeal/ wholewheat breadcrumbs	2 cups

1. Heat half the sunflower oil in a shallow non-stick frying pan (skillet). Add the onion and garlic and fry over a low heat for 5 minutes.
2. Stir in the tomato purée (paste), oregano or marjoram and black pepper.
3. Tip the mixture into the goblet of a liquidizer (blender) or food processor. Add the chickpeas (garbanzos) and most of the breadcrumbs – retaining about 2 tablespoons breadcrumbs for the coating. Process to a smooth paste.

4. Scoop the mixture out of the goblet and shape it into a sausage. Coat the surface with the remaining bread-crumbs.

5. Lightly oil a baking sheet and gently brush the roll with the remaining oil.

6. Bake the roll in a pre-heated oven set at 400°F/200°C/gas mark 6 for 30 minutes.

7. Serve hot. This dish goes well with onion gravy and fresh vegetables.

Note to Cooks

Can be frozen at stages 4 or 6.

PEANUTS SWEET AND SOUR

This recipe can also be used as a Between-Meal-Snack.

Serves 4
135 Calories ½ portion

Metric/Imperial		American
115g/4oz	button mushrooms	2 cups
10	spring onions/scallions	10
2 sticks	celery	2 stalks
1 medium	green/bell pepper	1 medium
1 medium	red/sweet pepper	1 medium
1 tbs	sunflower oil	1 tbs
115g/4oz	peanuts	¾ cup
115g/4oz	brown rice, cooked	⅔ cup

Dressing

1 tbs	freshly chopped root ginger	1 tbs
1 clove	garlic, crushed/minced	1 clove
1 slice	fresh pineapple	1 slice
1	lemon, zest and juice	1
2 tbs	soya/soy sauce	2 tbs

1. Wipe and thinly slice the mushrooms.
2. Trim, wash and slice the spring onions (scallions) diagonally into 2.5cm (1 in) pieces.
3. Slice the celery as described in stage 2.
4. Wash, de-seed and slice the peppers into 1.25 x 2.5cm (½ x 1 in) pieces.

5. Heat the oil in a wok or large non-stick shallow frying pan (skillet). Add the vegetables, nuts and rice and fry for 3 minutes. Stir well.
6. Put the dressing ingredients into the goblet of a liquidizer (blender) or food processor and blend. Pour the dressing over the stir-fry and serve at once.

Note to Cooks

Can be frozen.

TOFU AND MUSHROOM KEBABS

Metric/Imperial		American
225g/½ lb	firm tofu	½ lb
115g/4oz	button mushrooms	2 cups
2 tbs	soya/soy sauce	2 tbs
2 tbs	smooth peanut butter	2 tbs
1 tbs	chilli sauce	1 tbs

1. Cut the tofu into 2.5cm (1 in) cubes.
2. Wipe the mushrooms.
3. Mix the soya (soy) sauce, peanut butter and chilli sauce together in a basin. Add the tofu and mushrooms and stir gently to coat with the marinade.
4. Leave the mixture to stand for 1 hour.
5. Put the tofu and mushrooms on to skewers and grill (broil) under a moderate heat for 2 minutes on each side.
6. Serve hot. This dish goes well with savoury rice and a variety of side salads.

CARBOHYDRATE 'RICH' DISHES

POTATO CAKES

Serves 6
80 Calories ½ portion

Metric/Imperial		American
455g/1 lb	potatoes	1 lb
1 small	onion	1 small
2 cloves	garlic	2 cloves
2 tbs	freshly chopped parsley	2 tbs
	nutmeg, freshly grated	
2	eggs	2
55g/2oz	wholemeal/wholewheat flour	½ cup
2 tbs	sunflower oil	2 tbs

1. Scrub, peel and finely grate the potatoes.
2. Peel and grate the onion.
3. Peel and crush (mince) the garlic.
4. Put the potato, onion, garlic, parsley and nutmeg into a mixing bowl.
5. Lightly beat the eggs.
6. Add the eggs and flour to the potato mixture and stir to form a firm batter.
7. Heat half the oil in a non-stick shallow frying pan (skillet). Drop 6 tablespoons of mixture into the pan. Each cake should spread to a diameter of about 5cm (2 in). Cook over a moderate heat, turning the cakes over after 5 minutes to ensure even cooking on both

sides. Continue cooking for a further 5 minutes.

8. Drain on kitchen paper (paper towels). Keep the cakes warm and cook the remainder in exactly the same way using the rest of the oil.

9. Serve hot.

POTATO SALAD

This recipe can also be used as a Between-Meal-Snack.

Serves 4
90 Calories ½ portion

Metric/Imperial		American
455g/1 lb	baby new potatoes	1 lb
2	spring onions/scallions	2
1 clove	garlic	1 clove
2	hard-boiled eggs	2
60ml/2 fl oz	low calorie mayonnaise	¼ cup
2 tbs	freshly chopped chives	2 tbs

1. Boil the potatoes until they are fully cooked. Drain and allow to cool.
2. Trim, rinse and finely chop the spring onions (scallions).
3. Peel and crush (mince) the garlic.
4. Shell and chop the hard-boiled eggs.
5. Mix the potato, spring onions (scallions), garlic, chopped egg and mayonnaise together in a large mixing bowl.
6. Pile the mixture into a serving dish and serve sprinkled with the freshly chopped chives.

RÖSTI

Serves 4
75 Calories ½ portion

Metric/Imperial		American
455g/1 lb	waxy potatoes	1 lb
3 cloves	garlic	3 cloves
	freshly milled black pepper	
30g/1oz	polyunsaturated margarine	2 tbs
1 tbs	freshly chopped parsley	1 tbs

1. Scrub and boil the potatoes in their skins for 10 minutes. Drain thoroughly and leave to cool.
2. Peel and crush (mince) the garlic.
3. Grate the potato, including the skins, and pile it into a mixing bowl.
4. Fold in the garlic and pepper.
5. Melt half the fat in a shallow non-stick frying pan (skillet). Add the potato and pat down using a round bladed knife. Cook over a moderate heat for 10 minutes.
6. Position a flat plate over the pan and invert the pan so that the potato falls on to the plate.
7. Put the remaining fat in the pan. When the fat has melted slide the potato cake back into the pan and continue cooking for 10 minutes.
8. Slide the rösti on to a hot serving plate. Sprinkle with freshly chopped parsley and serve promptly.

COUSCOUS

Serves 4
145 Calories ½ portion

Metric/Imperial		American
1 small	onion	1 small
1 medium	green/bell pepper	1 medium
3 tbs	sunflower oil	3 tbs
115g/4oz	petit pois	⅔ cup
	ground cumin	
225g/½ lb	couscous	2 cups
285ml/½ pint	water	1⅛ cups
55g/2oz	sultanas/golden seedless raisins	⅓ cup
55g/2oz	flaked/slivered almonds, toasted	½ cup

1. Peel and dice the onion.
2. De-seed, rinse and dice the pepper.
3. Heat 1 tablespoon of the oil in a heavy based oven-proof pan. Add the onion and fry over a moderate heat for 5 minutes.
4. Add the pepper, peas and a pinch of cumin. Continue cooking for 2 more minutes
5. Rub the remaining oil into the couscous using the finger tips. Be sure to coat all the grains.
6. Bring the water to boiling point in a large pan. Add the couscous and simmer for about 8 to 10 minutes. Stir frequently to keep the grains separate.

7. Add the couscous to the onion mixture. Stir in the sultanas (golden seedless raisins) and toasted almonds.
8. Put the dish into a pre-heated oven set at 400°F/ 200°C/gas mark 6 for 10 minutes.
9. Serve really hot.

PASTA SALAD

This recipe can also be used as a Between-Meal-Snack. It is also a good salad to use as a 'take-away', packed into a lidded container.

Serves 4
115 Calories ½ portion

Metric/Imperial		American
225g/½ lb	wholemeal/wholewheat pasta shapes	4 cups
1 small	onion	1 small
1 clove	garlic	1 clove
30g/1oz	fresh basil leaves	1 cup
1 tbs	sunflower oil	1 tbs
4 tbs	tomato purée/paste	4 tbs

1. Cook the pasta according to packet instructions.
2. Peel and dice the onion.
3. Peel and crush (mince) the garlic.
4. Wash, drain and chop the basil.
5. Heat the oil in a non-stick pan. Add the onion and garlic and fry over a moderate heat to soften the onion.
6. Stir in the freshly chopped basil and the tomato purée (paste).
7. Mix the hot pasta with the onion mixture and leave to cool.
8. Serve chilled.

PILAU RICE

Serves 4
115 Calories ½ portion

Metric/Imperial		American
1 medium	onion	1 medium
15g/½ oz	polyunsaturated margarine	1 tbs
225g/½ lb	brown rice	1 cup
570ml/1 pint	water	2½ cups
¼ tsp	cumin seeds	¼ tsp
1	cardamom pod	1
1	bay leaf	1
1 stick	cinnamon	1 stick

1. Peel and finely slice the onion.
2. Melt the margarine in a heavy based pan. Add the onion and fry over a moderate heat until the onion has softened.
3. Stir in the rice and ensure that all the grains are coated with the fat.
4. Add the water and bring to boiling point. Meanwhile crush the cumin seeds and cardamom pod using a pestle and mortar.
5. Add the bay leaf and spices to the rice and simmer with the lid on the pan for approximately 40 minutes.
6. Remove the bay leaf and cinnamon stick.
7. Pile the rice into a hot serving dish and serve without delay.

Note to Cooks
Can be frozen.

TABBOULEH

A very refreshing dish to serve with salads. This recipe can also be used as a Between-Meal-Snack.

Serves 4
115 Calories ½ portion

Metric/Imperial		American
170g/6oz	bulgar wheat	1 cup
20	spring onions/scallions	20
2 tbs	sunflower oil	2 tbs
1 tbs	fresh lemon juice	1 tbs
55g/2oz	freshly chopped mint	2 cups
55g/2oz	freshly chopped parsley	2 cups

1. Put the bulgar wheat in a large basin. Add enough cold water to cover the grains. Leave to stand for 1 hour.
2. Trim, rinse, drain and chop the spring onions (scallions) finely.
3. Mix the oil and lemon juice together in a small basin.
4. Drain any excess liquid from the bulgar wheat and mix the grains with the spring onions (scallions), freshly chopped herbs and the oil and lemon dressing.
5. Pile the mixture into a serving dish and chill for 1 hour.
6. Serve cold.

VEGETABLE RICE

Serves 4
125 Calories ½ portion

Metric/Imperial		*American*
1 tbs	sunflower oil	1 tbs
225g/½ lb	brown rice	1 cup
1 tbs	tomato purée/paste	1 tbs
570ml/1 pint	vegetable stock	2½ cups
55g/2oz	frozen peas	⅓ cup
55g/2oz	carrot, diced	⅓ cup
55g/2oz	frozen sweetcorn kernels	⅓ cup

1. Pour the oil into a heavy based pan. Put over a moderate heat and add the rice. Fry the mixture for 2 minutes and stir constantly.
2. Add the tomato purée (paste) and stir into the rice.
3. Pour the vegetable stock into the pan. Bring to boiling point and simmer with the lid on the pan for 30 minutes.
4. Add the vegetables and continue cooking for 10 minutes.
5. Pile the mixture into a hot serving dish and serve at once.

Note to Cooks

Can be frozen.

CARROTS AND CAPERS

Serves 4
30 Calories ½ portion

Metric/Imperial		American
455g/1 lb	young carrots	1 lb
1 clove	garlic	1 clove
1 tbs	sunflower oil	1 tbs
30g/1oz	freshly chopped parsley	1 cup
140ml/¼ pint	vegetable stock	⅔ cup
1 tbs	capers	1 tbs

1. Peel, scrape, rinse and cut the carrots into finger size pieces.
2. Peel and crush (mince) the garlic.
3. Heat the oil in a heavy based pan. Add the garlic and cook over a moderate heat until the garlic turns golden. Add the carrots and parsley and stir fry for 2 minutes.
4. Add the stock and simmer for 12 to 15 minutes. When the water has evaporated allow the carrots to lightly brown.
5. Add the capers and continue cooking for 2 minutes.
6. Serve at once.

Note to Cooks

Can be frozen.

FRENCH/SNAP BEANS WITH GARLIC

Serves 4
20 Calories ½ portion

Metric/Imperial		American
455g/1 lb	French/snap beans	1 lb
5 cloves	garlic	5 cloves
15g/½ oz	polyunsaturated margarine	1 tbs
2 tbs	freshly chopped parsley	2 tbs

1. Top and tail the beans; rinse under cold running water and drain thoroughly.
2. Peel and crush (mince) the garlic.
3. Cook the beans with just enough water to cover for 7 minutes and drain well.
4. Heat the margarine in a shallow non-stick frying pan (skillet) and add the garlic. Fry over a low heat for 30 seconds to soften the garlic.
5. Add the beans and stir thoroughly for 1 minute.
6. Serve hot sprinkled with the fresh parsley.

Note to Cooks

Can be frozen.

RATATOUILLE

This dish is delicious hot or cold.

Serves 4
40 Calories ½ portion

Metric/Imperial		American
1 medium	aubergine/eggplant	1 medium
1 tbs	salt	1 tbs
455g/1 lb	tomatoes	1 lb
225g/½ lb	courgettes/zucchini	½ lb
1 medium	green/bell pepper	1 medium
1	Spanish onion	1
1 clove	garlic	1 clove
30g/1oz	fresh basil leaves	1 cup
1 tbs	sunflower oil	1 tbs

1. Trim the stalk from the aubergine (eggplant) and cut the vegetable into 1cm (½ in) slices. Spread the slices on a flat dish and sprinkle with salt. Leave for 1 hour. Wash thoroughly under cold running water and drain well.
2. Skin, de-seed and chop the tomatoes.
3. Trim, wash and cut the courgettes (zucchini) into 1cm (½ in) slices.
4. De-seed, rinse and cut the pepper into 5mm (¼ in) strips.
5. Peel and thinly slice the onion.
6. Peel and crush (mince) the garlic.
7. Wash the fresh basil and drain well.

8. Heat the oil in a heavy based pan. Add all the vegetables and basil. Stir gently, then leave to simmer with the lid on the pan for 45 minutes.

9. Serve hot or cold.

Note to Cooks

Can be frozen.

RED CABBAGE

Serves 4
40 Calories ½ portion

Metric/Imperial		*American*
455g/1 lb	red cabbage	1 lb
1 small	onion	1 small
2	eating apples	2
1 tbs	sunflower oil	1 tbs
1 tbs	lemon juice	1 tbs
¼ tsp	powdered cloves	¼ tsp
2 tbs	water	2 tbs

1. Trim and cut the cabbage into quarters. Remove the stalk and separate the leaves. Wash under cold running water and drain thoroughly. Shred the leaves, using a sharp stainless steel knife or a food processor with shredder attachment.
2. Peel and thinly slice the onion.
3. Peel, core and slice the apples.
4. Heat the oil in a heavy based pan. Add the onion and fry over a low heat to soften but not to brown the onion.
5. Add the red cabbage, apples, lemon juice, powdered cloves and water. Stir thoroughly.
6. Put the lid on the pan and leave to simmer for 45 minutes. Stir periodically to prevent sticking.
7. Serve hot.

Note to Cooks

Can be frozen.

SPINACH AND MUSHROOMS

Serves 4
75 Calories ½ portion

Metric/Imperial		*American*
455g/1 lb	frozen spinach	1 lb
225g/½ lb	mushrooms	4 cups
30g/1oz	polyunsaturated margarine	2 tbs
55g/2oz	Gruyère cheese, grated	½ cup

1. Cook the spinach according to packet instructions and chop coarsely.
2. Wipe the mushrooms and slice very finely.
3. Put half the margarine into a pan over a moderate heat. Add the spinach and stir continually for 5 minutes.
4. Put the remaining margarine into another pan over a moderate heat and add the mushrooms. Fry for about 3 minutes stirring constantly.
5. Mix the spinach and mushrooms together and spoon the mixture into a lightly greased ovenproof dish.
6. Sprinkle the cheese over the top of the vegetable mixture.
7. Bake for 15 minutes in a pre-heated oven set at 375°F/190°C/gas mark 5.
8. Serve hot.

Note to Cooks

Can be frozen at stages 6 or 7.

VEGETABLE STIR FRY

Serves 4
75 Calories ½ portion

Metric/Imperial		*American*
455g/1 lb	mangetout/snow peas	1 lb
1 bulb	fennel	1 bulb
4 sticks	celery	4 stalks
8	spring onions/scallions	8
2 tbs	freshly chopped ginger root	2 tbs
1 tbs	sunflower oil	1 tbs
1 tsp	honey	1 tsp
1 tbs	soya/soy sauce	1 tbs
1 tsp	wine vinegar	1 tsp

1. Trim the mangetout (snow peas) and blanch in boiling water for 1 minute. Plunge into cold water and drain thoroughly.
2. Separate the fennel, rinse and cut into thin 5mm (¼ in) wide strips.
3. Scrub, string and cut the celery into 5mm (¼ in) wide strips.
4. Trim, rinse and cut the spring onions (scallions) into 2.5cm (1 in) lengths.
5. Heat the oil in a wok or shallow non-stick frying pan (skillet). Add the fennel, celery, spring onions (scallions) and ginger. Stir fry over a moderate heat for 5 minutes.
6. Add the mangetout (snow peas) and cook for 2 more minutes.

PMS

7. Add the honey, soya (soy) sauce and wine vinegar. Stir thoroughly and cook for 1 minute. Serve without delay.

Note to Cooks

Can be frozen.

BEETROOT/BEET SALAD

Serves 4
40 Calories ½ portion

Metric/Imperial		American
455g/1 lb	boiled beetroot/beet	1 lb
1 tbs	fresh lemon juice	1 tbs
1 tbs	sunflower oil	1 tbs
285ml/½ pint	plain low fat yogurt	1⅓ cups
2 tbs	freshly chopped parsley	2 tbs

1. Trim the beetroot (beet), dice and put into a mixing bowl.
2. Mix the lemon juice and oil together in a basin. Add the yogurt and beat well.
3. Pour the dressing over the beetroot (beet) and gently fold the mixture together.
4. Tip the salad into a serving dish and sprinkle with the parsley.
5. Serve chilled.

FRUITY CARROT SALAD

Serves 4
55 Calories ½ portion

Metric/Imperial		American
455g/1 lb	carrots	1 lb
1 medium	orange	1 medium
115g/4oz	sultanas/golden seedless raisins	⅔ cup
1 tbs	freshly grated ginger root	1 tbs

1. Peel or scrape, rinse and grate the carrots and put them into a mixing bowl.
2. Segment the orange over the mixing bowl so that the juice falls on to the carrots. Add the orange segments to the carrots.
3. Add the sultanas (golden seedless raisins) and ginger to the mixture. Gently fold the ingredients together.
4. Serve chilled.

GREEN SALAD WITH MINT

Serves 4
5 Calories ½ portion

Metric/Imperial		American
1	cos/romaine lettuce	1
1 medium	green/bell pepper	1 medium
55g/2oz	watercress	2 cups
30g/1oz	fresh mint leaves	1 cup

1. Separate the lettuce leaves, wash and drain thoroughly. Shred, using a sharp knife.
2. De-seed, rinse and cut the pepper into 5mm (¼ in) strips.
3. Wash and drain the watercress and mint.
4. Put all the ingredients into a large serving bowl and fold the mixture together.
5. Serve at once.

MINTY CUCUMBER SALAD

Metric/Imperial		American
1 medium	cucumber	1 medium
1 clove	garlic	1 clove
15g/½ oz	freshly chopped mint	½ cup
140ml/¼ pint	plain low fat yogurt	⅔ cup
6 sprigs	fresh mint	6 sprigs

1. Wash and slice the cucumber and arrange on a flat plate.
2. Peel and crush (mince) the garlic.
3. Mix the garlic, mint and yogurt together in a small basin.
4. Pour the dressing over the cucumber and garnish with sprigs of fresh mint.

MUSHROOM SALAD

Serves 4
25 Calories ½ portion

Metric/Imperial		American
455g/1 lb	button mushrooms	1 lb
2 cloves	garlic	2 cloves
1 tbs	sunflower oil	1 tbs
2 tsps	fresh lemon juice	2 tsps
30g/1oz	freshly chopped parsley	1 cup

1. Wipe the mushrooms and slice thinly.
2. Peel and crush (mince) the garlic.
3. Heat the oil in a shallow non-stick frying pan (skillet). Add the garlic and mushrooms and cook over a moderate heat for 5 minutes.
4. Add the lemon juice and stir thoroughly over the heat for 1 more minute.
5. Pour the mixture into a serving dish. Allow to cool and chill for 1 hour.
6. Serve sprinkled with the freshly chopped parsley.

TOMATO SALAD WITH BASIL

Serves 4
40 Calories ½ portion

Metric/Imperial		American
455g/1 lb	firm salad tomatoes	1 lb
55g/2oz	fresh basil leaves	2 cups
2 tbs	sunflower oil	2 tbs
1 tbs	lemon juice	1 tbs
¼ tsp	mustard powder	¼ tsp

1. Trim, wash and drain and slice the tomatoes very thinly.
2. Wash, drain and chop the fresh basil.
3. Pour the oil and lemon juice into a small bottle. Add the mustard and shake vigorously.
4. Arrange the tomatoes on a flat serving dish. Sprinkle with the chopped basil and drizzle the salad dressing evenly over the top.
5. Serve cold.

SWEETS

BANANA SURPRISE

Serves 6
90 Calories ½ portion

Metric/Imperial		American
4 large	bananas	4 large
55g/2oz	chopped dates	⅓ cup
55g/2oz	chopped dried apricots	⅓ cup
55g/2oz	sultanas/golden seedless raisins	⅓ cup
55g/2oz	chopped almonds	½ cup

1. Peel the bananas and mash in a large mixing bowl.
2. Add the fruit and nuts and stir thoroughly.
3. Spread the mixture in a shallow freezer tray or Swiss roll (jelly roll) tin. Cover with aluminium foil and freeze for 3 hours.
4. Serve in individual dishes.

DATE AND BANANA PUDDING

Serves 4
180 Calories ½ portion

Metric/Imperial		American
4 large	bananas	4 large
1 tbs	freshly squeezed lemon juice	1 tbs
285g/10oz	stoned/pitted dried dates	2 cups
285ml/½ pint	fromage frais	1⅓ cups
2 tbs	wheatgerm	2 tbs

1. Peel the bananas, slice and put into a mixing bowl. Add the lemon juice and gently fold the mixture to coat the slices with the lemon juice.
2. Cut the dates into halves.
3. Arrange layers of the bananas and dates in a serving dish until all the fruit is used up.
4. Top with the fromage frais and chill for 30 minutes.
5. Sprinkle with the wheatgerm and serve.

DRIED FRUIT COMPOTE

Serves 4
75 Calories ½ portion

Metric/Imperial		American
70g/2½oz	dried figs	½ cup
70g/2½oz	dried apricots	½ cup
70g/2½oz	dried prunes	½ cup
70g/2½oz	dried apple	½ cup
285ml/½ pint	apple juice	1⅛ cups

1. Put the dried fruit into a bowl with the apple juice and leave covered in the refrigerator overnight.
2. Serve chilled.

RED FRUIT SALAD

Serves 4
15 Calories ½ portion

Metric/Imperial		American
225g/½ lb	strawberries	2 cups
225g/½ lb	raspberries	2 cups
115g/4oz	red currants	1 cup
90ml/3 fl oz	unsweetened cranberry juice	⅓ cup

1. Remove any stems and leaves from the fruit and wash gently in a colander under cold running water.
2. Put the fruit into a serving bowl and stir in the cranberry juice.
3. Chill for 30 minutes.

YOGURT TREAT

Serves 4
60 Calories ½ portion

Metric/Imperial		American
4 medium	bananas	4 medium
140ml/¼ pint	plain low fat yogurt	⅔ cup
¼ tsp	vanilla essence	¼ tsp
30g/1oz	flaked/slivered almonds, toasted	¼ cup

1. Peel the bananas and mash them in a large mixing bowl.
2. Add the yogurt and vanilla essence and stir thoroughly.
3. Pour the mixture into a shallow freezer tray or Swiss roll (jelly roll) tin. Cover with aluminium foil and freeze for 3 hours.
4. Serve in individual dishes and sprinkle with the toasted almonds.

APPLE CRUNCH

Serves 4
150 Calories ½ portion

Metric/Imperial		American
455g/1 lb	cooking apples	1 lb
½ small	lemon, juice of	½ small
2 tbs	water	2 tbs
55g/2oz	polyunsaturated margarine	¼ cup
30g/1oz	brown sugar	2 tbs
55g/2oz	flaked/slivered almonds	½ cup
¼ tsp	mixed spice	¼ tsp
115g/4oz	fresh wholemeal/ wholewheat breadcrumbs	2 cups

1. Peel, core and slice the apples.
2. Put the apples into a pan with the lemon juice and water. Cook over a moderate heat for 10 minutes.
3. Melt the margarine in a shallow non-stick frying pan (skillet) over a moderate heat. Add the sugar, almonds, mixed spice and breadcrumbs. Stir the mixture thoroughly.
4. Pour the lightly stewed apple into a pie dish and top with the breadcrumb mixture.
5. Bake in a pre-heated oven set at 350°F/180°C/gas mark 4 for 30 minutes.
6. Serve hot or cold.

BREAD AND SULTANA/RAISIN PUDDING

Serves 4
115 Calories ½ portion

Metric/Imperial		American
30g/1oz	polyunsaturated margarine	2 tbs
4 slices	wholemeal/wholewheat bread	4 slices
85g/3oz	sultanas/golden seedless raisins	½ cup
1	egg	1
285ml/½ pint	semi-skimmed/low fat milk	1⅓ cups
	freshly grated nutmeg	

1. Spread the fat on the slices of bread and cut the bread into 2.5cm (1 in) squares.
2. Arrange half the bread on the base of a lightly greased 570ml (1 pint) pie dish.
3. Sprinkle the fruit over the top, then cover with the remaining bread.
4. Beat the egg with 2 tablespoons of the milk, in a basin.
5. Heat the remaining milk until it steams, then stir this into the egg mixture to form a custard.
6. Strain the custard over the bread mixture and sprinkle with freshly grated nutmeg.
7. Bake in a pre-heated oven set at 350°F/180°C/gas mark 4 for 35 minutes.

PINEAPPLE KEBABS

Serves 4
30 Calories ½ portion

Metric/Imperial		American
1 medium	pineapple	1 medium
1 tbs	stem ginger syrup	1 tbs
1 tbs	finely chopped stem ginger	1 tbs

1. Cut off the pineapple crown, quarter the fruit lengthways and remove the core. Separate fruit from rind and cut into 2.5cm (1 in) cubes.
2. Mix the syrup and chopped stem ginger together in a basin.
3. Put the pineapple chunks into the basin and gently fold the ingredients together so that the flavours mingle.
4. Cover and leave to stand for about 8 hours.
5. Thread the fruit on to 4 kebab skewers and cook under a moderate grill (broiler) for 5 minutes, turning frequently.
6. Serve without delay.

RICE DESSERT

Serves 4
65 Calories ½ portion

Metric/Imperial		American
55g/2oz	pudding rice	¼ cup
1 tbs	caster sugar	1 tbs
570ml/1 pint	semi-skimmed/low fat milk	2½ cups
1 tsp	vanilla essence	1 tsp
	freshly grated nutmeg	

1. Put the rice into a heavy based pan with the sugar and milk.
2. Cook over a low heat and stir continuously until the mixture bubbles.
3. Put the lid on the pan and leave to simmer for about 30 minutes.
4. Remove the pan from the heat and stir in the vanilla essence.
5. Spoon the mixture into individual serving dishes. Serve hot or cold sprinkled with the freshly grated nutmeg.

Emergency snacks

DIGESTIVE BISCUITS/ GRAHAM CRACKERS

This recipe can also be used as a Between-Meal-Snack.

Makes 24
65 Calories each

Metric/Imperial		American
170g/6oz	wholemeal/wholewheat flour	1½ cups
1 tsp	baking powder/soda	1 tsp
55g/2oz	fine oatmeal	½ cup
85g/3oz	polyunsaturated margarine	⅓ cup
30g/1oz	soft brown sugar	2 tbs
4 tbs	semi-skimmed/low fat milk	4 tbs
1 tbs	sesame seeds	1 tbs

1. Sift (strain) the flour and baking powder (soda) into a large mixing bowl. Tip any remaining bran into the bowl.

2. Add the oatmeal and margarine. Rub in the fat until the mixture looks like breadcrumbs.
3. Add the sugar and milk and stir into a dough.
4. Roll the dough out very thinly on a floured work surface. Cut into 6cm (2½ in) rounds. Pierce the surface of the raw biscuits (cookies) with a fork. Then brush with water and sprinkle with the sesame seeds. Carefully lift the biscuits (cookies) on to 2 non-stick or lightly greased baking sheets.
5. Bake in a pre-heated oven set at 375°F/190°C/gas mark 5 for about 15 minutes.
6. Lift the biscuits (cookies) on to a cooling rack.
7. Store in an airtight container for up to 1 week.

PEANUT BISCUITS/COOKIES

This recipe can also be used as a Between-Meal-Snack.

Makes 12
95 Calories each

Metric/Imperial		American
55g/2oz	polyunsaturated margarine	¼ cup
30g/1oz	soft brown sugar	2 tbs
55g/2oz	chopped roasted salted peanuts	½ cup
85g/3oz	self-raising/rising brown flour	¾ cup
½ tsp	mixed spice	½ tsp
1 tbs	fresh orange juice	1 tbs

1. Cream the fat and sugar together in a large mixing bowl until the mixture is fluffy.
2. Add the peanuts and sift (strain) the flour and spice into the bowl. Tip any remaining bran into the bowl.
3. Stir in the orange juice and mix well.
4. Divide the mixture into 12 pieces and form into balls.
5. Put the balls on to a non-stick or lightly greased baking sheet and flatten them using a rolling pin.
6. Bake in a pre-heated oven set at 350°F/180°C/gas mark 4 for about 10 minutes.
7. Leave the biscuits (cookies) on the tray for 15 minutes. Then lift them on to a cooling rack.
8. Store in an airtight container for up to 1 week.

ALL-BRAN CAKE

This recipe can also be used as a Between-Meal-Snack.

Cuts into 18 slices
110 Calories a slice

Metric/Imperial		American
115g/4oz	All-Bran	1½ cups
85g/3oz	caster sugar	½ cup
340g/¾ lb	mixed dried fruit	2 cups
285ml/½ pint	semi-skimmed/low fat milk	1⅓ cups
115g/4oz	self-raising/rising brown flour	1 cup

1. Put the All-Bran, sugar, dried fruit and milk into a large mixing bowl. Stir the mixture thoroughly and leave to stand for 30 minutes.
2. Sift (strain) the flour into the mixture and tip in any remaining bran. Mix well.
3. Pour the cake mixture into a non-stick or lightly greased and lined 900g (2 lb) loaf tin.
4. Bake in a pre-heated oven set at 350°F/180°C/gas mark 4 for about 1 hour.
5. Leave the cake to stand for 15 minutes; then turn it on to a cooling rack.
6. When cold, wrap in aluminium foil and keep for up to 1 week.

Note to Cooks

Can be frozen.

BANANA AND WALNUT/
ENGLISH WALNUT CAKE

This recipe can also be used as a Between-Meal-Snack.

12 slices
215 Calories a slice

Metric/Imperial		American
200g/7oz	wholemeal self-raising/ wholewheat self-rising flour	1¾ cups
½ tsp	mixed spice	½ tsp
115g/4oz	polyunsaturated margarine	½ cup
115g/4oz	chopped walnuts/English walnuts	¾ cup
85g/3oz	chopped stoned/pitted raisins	½ cup
2 small	ripe bananas, mashed	2 small
1 tbs	thin honey	1 tbs
2	eggs, lightly beaten	2

1. Sift (strain) the flour and spice into a large mixing bowl. Tip in bran remaining in the sieve (strainer).
2. Add the margarine and rub into the flour until the mixture looks like fine breadcrumbs.
3. Add the walnuts (English walnuts) and raisins and stir well.
4. Add the bananas, honey and eggs and mix thoroughly.
5. Pour the cake mixture into a non-stick or lightly greased and lined 455g (1 lb) loaf tin.

6. Bake in a pre-heated oven set at 350°F/180°C/gas mark 4 for about 1 hour.
7. Leave the cake to stand for 15 minutes, then turn it on to a cooling rack.
8. Wrap in aluminium foil and keep for up to 1 week.

Note to Cooks

Can be frozen.

DATE AND BRAZIL NUT CAKE

This recipe can also be used as a Between-Meal-Snack.

18 slices
160 Calories a slice

Metric/Imperial		American
255g/9oz	wholemeal/wholewheat flour	2¼ cups
2 tsps	baking powder/soda	2 tsps
140g/5oz	chopped brazil nuts	1 cup
170g/6oz	chopped dried dates	1 cup
90ml/3 fl oz	sunflower oil	⅓ cup
200ml/⅓ pint	water	¾ cup

1. Sift (strain) the flour and baking powder (soda) into a large mixing bowl. Tip any remaining bran into the bowl.
2. Add the nuts and a third of the dates.
3. Put the remaining dates into the goblet of a liquidizer (blender) or food processor with the oil and water. Process the mixture until it looks like syrup.
4. Pour the liquid onto the ingredients in the mixing bowl and stir thoroughly.
5. Spoon the cake mixture into a non-stick or lightly greased and lined 15cm (6 in) round cake tin or 900g (2 lb) loaf tin.
6. Bake in a pre-heated oven set at 350°F/180°C/gas mark 4 for about 1 hour.

7. Leave the cake to stand for 15 minutes and then turn it on to a cooling rack.
8. When cold, wrap in aluminium foil and keep for up to 1 week.

Note to Cooks

Can be frozen.

Further Reading

PREMENSTRUAL SYNDROME

Dalton, K., *Premenstrual Syndrome and Progesterone Therapy* 2nd Edition, William Heinemann, Medical Books, 1984.

Dalton, K., *Once a Month*, 5th Edition, Fontana/HarperCollins, 1991.

Dalton, K., *Premenstrual Syndrome goes to Court*, Peter Andrew Publishing Company, Droitwich, 1990.

Dalton, K., *Premenstrual Syndrome Illustrated*, Peter Andrew Publishing Company, Droitwich, 1990.

Dalton, K. and Holton, D., *PMS The Essential Guide to Treatment Options*, Thorsons, 1994.

DIET

Coultate, T., and Davies, J., *Food: The Definitive Guide*, Royal Society of Chemistry, 1994.

Holton, W., *Can Diet Help your PMS?* PMS Help, P.O. Box 160, St Albans, Herts, AL1 4UQ.

Useful Addresses

PMS Help
PO Box 160
St Albans
Herts AL1 4UQ

Membership of PMS Help means that you will receive a
quarterly bulletin and be kept up to date on research on
PMS. You will also be in contact with fellow-sufferers
and experts who have an interest in the condition. The
group is growing from strength to strength and warmly
welcomes new members. I thoroughly recommend join-
ing PMS Help if you or a member of your family suffer
from PMS.

General Index

adrenalin 7
alcohol 24
anti-depressants 12

blood sugar
  diet 9
  levels 8
  regulation 7
bromocriptine 12

caffeine 26
carbohydrate 9
causes 5, 6, 7, 8
complex carbohydrate 9

definition 3
diagnosis 5
diet
  alcoholic drinks 25
  caffeinated beverages 26

carbohydrate 9
complex carbohydrate
  21
fat 19, 20, 21
salt 23
sugar 17
water 25
diuretics 12

eating pattern 26–34
evening primrose oil
  14–15

fat 19–21

hormones
  adrenalin 7
  insulin 7
  progesterone 7
  prolactin 7

hormone therapy
  progesterone implants
    11
  progesterone injections
    11
  progesterone
    suppositories 11
  progestogens 12

incidence 1
insulin 6

lifestyle 15–16

meal planning 29–32
meal spacing 10

nutritional supplements
  evening primrose oil 14
  vitamin B$_6$ 13

pharmacological
    preparations
  anti-depressants 13

bromocriptine 12
diuretics 12
nutritional supplements
    13–14
progesterone 7
progesterone implants 11
progesterone injections
    11
progesterone receptors 7
progesterone suppositories
    11
progestogens 12
prolactin 8
prostaglandins 8
psychotherapy 15

salt 3, 4, 5
sugar 17

vitamin B$_6$ 13–14

water 25

Recipe Index

All-Bran cake 194
almond potato cakes 50
apple crunch 187
avocado with fruit 117

bacon
   baked bean burgers 52
   breakfast pancakes/
     crêpes 38
   egg and bacon burgers
     44
   jacket potato, bacon
     and sweetcorn filling
     86
   mushroom caps with
     savoury filling 127
   potato salad with ham
     66
   rösti, bacon and tomato
     topping 90

scramble on toast, bacon
   flavoured 100
baked bean burgers 52
banana and walnut/
   English walnut cake
   195
banana surprise 182
bean dip 63
bean soup 107
beef
   beefburgers 105
   chilli-con-carne 145
beetroot/beet salad 176
biscuits
   digestive biscuits/
     graham crackers 191
   oaty biscuits/cookies
     77
   peanut biscuits/cookies
     193

bread(s)
  apple crunch 187
  baked bean burgers 52
  bran muffins 35
  bread and sultana/raisin
    pudding 188
  brunch bread 79
  cashew and lentil loaf
    69
  cheese scones 54
  cheese and vegetable
    bake 133
  cheesy loaf 71
  cheesy pudding 94
  chickpea/garbanzo roast
    153
  crab bites 56
  falafel 109
  garlic bites 58
  Glamorgan sausages 95
  lentil burgers 114
  mushroom caps with
    savoury filling 127
  pitta pockets 88
  Stilton loaf 73
  tea bread 84
bread and sultana/raisin
    pudding 188
breakfast cereals
  All-Bran cake 194

  brunch bread 79
  cheesy loaf 71
  crunchy brek 40
  muesli 48
breakfast cocktail 37
  breakfast pancakes/
    crêpes 38
brunch bread 79
cakes
  All-Bran cake 194
  banana and walnut/
    English walnut cake
    195
carrot and hazelnut cake
    81
  date and brazil nut cake
    197
  fruit and nut bites 75
  muesli bars 76
carrot and hazelnut cake
    81
carrots and capers 168
cashew and lentil loaf 69
cheese
  cheese and mushroom
    pâté 92
  cheese and vegetable
    bake 133
  cheese scones 54
  cheesy loaf 71

cheesy pudding 94
egg and spinach cake
    138
Glamorgan sausages 95
jacket potato, cheese
    and mango chutney
    filling 86
pesto 135
pitta pocket, feta cheese,
    tomato and onion
    filling 88
potato and spinach
    cakes 59
potato pizza 97
rösti, Swiss cheese
    topping 91
scrambles on toast
    cheese flavoured 100
spinach and mushrooms
    173
Stilton loaf 73
cheesy pudding 94
chicken
    chicken and tarragon
        salad 152
    chicken with fruit and
        nuts 150
    jacket potato, chicken,
        yogurt and mint
        filling 87

vegetable rice with
    chicken 68
chickpea/garbanzo roast
    153
chilli-con-carne 145
cookies
    digestive biscuits/
        graham crackers 191
    oaty biscuits/cookies 77
    peanut biscuits/cookies
        193
couscous 162
crab bites 56
crunchy brek 40

date and banana pudding
    188
date and brazil nut cake
    197
devilled kidneys 42
digestive biscuits/graham
    crackers 191
dips
    bean dip 63
    gingery vegetable dip
        131
    hummus 113
    peanut dip 64
    potato dip 130
dried fruit compôte 184

eggs
  breakfast pancakes/
    crêpes 38
  cheesy pudding 94
  egg and bacon burgers
    44
  egg and spinach cake
    138
  egg curry 136
  pitta pocket, egg,
    mustard and cress
    and mayonnaise
    filling 88
  potato cakes 158
  potato omelette Persian
    style 99
  potato salad 160
  rösti, poached egg and
    parsley topping 90
  Scotch eggs 106
  scrambles on toast
    100
  toad-in-the-hole 149

falafel 109
fish
  crab bites 56
  fish pie 140
  herring in apple and
    oatmeal 46

jacket potato, tuna and
  mayonnaise filling 87
kedgeree 47
kipper pâté 102
pasta salad with tuna
  65
pitta pocket, tuna,
  cucumber and yogurt
  filling 89
potato topped with
  mackerel 142
salmon fish cakes 103
sardine bake – Italian
  style 143
scramble on toast,
  smoked haddock and
  parsley flavoured
  100
French/snap beans with
  garlic 169
fruit
  All-Bran cake 194
  apple crunch 187
  avocado with fruit 117
  banana and walnut/
    English walnut cake
    195
  banana surprise 182
  bread and sultana/raisin
    pudding 188

breakfast cocktail 37

brunch bread 79

chicken with fruit and
  nuts 150

couscous 162

crunchy brek 40

date and banana
  pudding 188

date and brazil nut cake
  197

dried fruit compôte 184

fruit and nut bites 75

fruit and nut spread 83

fruity carrot salad 177

herring in apple and
  oatmeal 46

jacket potato, sausage,
  apple and sage filling
  87

lamb with dried fruit
  147

muesli 48

muesli bars 76

peanut dip 64

peanuts sweet and sour
  155

pineapple kebabs 189

red cabbage 172

red fruit salad 185

tangy carrot soup 129

tea bread 84

garlic bites 58

gazpacho 119

gingery vegetable dip 131

Glamorgan sausages 95

green salad with mint 178

herring in apple and
  oatmeal 46

hummus 113

jacket potatoes 86

kedgeree 47

kipper pâté 102

lamb with dried fruit 147

lentil burgers 114

lentil pâté 121

lentil soup 123

minty cucumber salad 179

minty lentil salad 115

muesli 48

muesli bars 76

mushroom caps with
  savoury filling 127

mushroom pâté 125

mushroom salad 180

nuts
almond potato cake 50
banana and walnut/
    English walnut cake
    195
brunch bread 79
carrot and hazelnut cake
    81
cashew and lentil loaf
    69
chicken with fruit and
    nuts 150
crunchy brek 40
couscous 162
date and brazil nut cake
    197
fruit and nut bites 75
fruit and nut spread 83
muesli 48
peanut biscuits/cookies
    193
peanut dip 64
peanuts sweet and sour
    155
potato and parsnip
    cakes 59
Stilton loaf 73
tabbouleh with peanuts
    67
yogurt treat 186

oaty biscuits/cookies 77

pasta
pesto 135
pasta salad 164
pasta salad with tuna 65
peanut biscuits/cookies
    193
peanut dip 64
peanuts sweet and sour
    155
pesto 135
pilau rice 165
pitta pockets 88
potatoes
almond potato cakes
    50
egg and bacon burgers
    44
fish pie 140
gingery vegetable dip
    131
jacket potatoes 86
lentil pâté 121
potato and parsnip
    cakes 59
potato and spinach
    cakes 61
potato cakes 158
potato dip 130

potato omelette Persian style 99
potato pizza 97
potato salad 160
potato salad with ham 66
potato topped with mackerel 142
rösti 161
rösti meals 90
salmon fishcakes 103
sardine bake – Italian style 143
potato and parsnip cakes 59
potato and spinach cakes 61
potato cakes 158
potato dip 130
potato omelette Persian style 99
potato pizza 97
potato salad 160
potato salad with ham 66
potato topped with mackerel 142
pulses
baked bean burgers 52
bean dip 63
bean soup 107

cashew and lentil loaf 69
chickpea/garbanzo roast 153
chilli-con-carne 145
falafel 109
hummus 113
lentil burgers 114
lentil pâté 121
lentil salad 115
lentil soup 123
rösti sausage and beans topping 90
spicy lentil soup 111
ratatouille 170
red cabbage 172
red fruit salad 185
rice
egg and spinach cake 138
kedgeree 47
peanuts sweet and sour 155
pilau rice 165
rice dessert 190
vegetable rice 167
vegetable rice with chicken 68
rice dessert 190
rösti 161

rösti meals 90

salads
  beetroot/beet salad 176
  chicken and tarragon
    salad 152
  fruity carrot salad 177
  green salad with mint
    178
  lentil salad 115
  minty cucumber salad
    179
  mushroom salad 180
  pasta salad 164
  pasta salad with tuna
    65
  potato salad 160
  potato salad with ham 66
  tabbouleh 166
  tabbouleh with peanuts
    67
  tomato salad with basil
    181
salmon fish cakes 103
sardine bake – Italian style
  143
sausages
  jacket potato, sausage,
    apple and sage filling
    87

rösti, sausage and beans
  topping 90
Scotch eggs 106
spicy sausages 49
toad-in-the-hole 149
Scotch eggs 106
scrambles on toast 100
soups
  bean soup 107
  gazpacho 119
  lentil soup 123
  spicy lentil soup 111
  tangy carrot soup 129
spicy lentil soup 111
spicy sausages 49
spinach and mushrooms
  173
spreads
  fruit and nut spread 83
  kipper pâté 102
  lentil pâté 121
  mushroom pâté 125
Stilton loaf 73
sweet and sour shallots
  132

tabbouleh 166
tabbouleh with peanuts
  67
tangy carrot soup 129

tea bread 84
toad-in-the-hole 149
tofu
    pitta pocket, smoked
        tofu, lettuce and
        watercress filling 88
    rösti, smoked tofu and
        mushroom topping
        90
    tofu and mushroom
        kebabs 157
tomato salad with basil
    181

vegetables
    carrots and capers 168
    French/snap beans with
        garlic 169
    ratatouille 170
    red cabbage 172
    spinach and mushrooms
        173
    sweet and sour shallots
        132

vegetable stir fry 174
vegetable rice 167
vegetable rice with
    chicken 68
vegetable stir fry 174

yogurt
    beetroot/beet salad 176
    breakfast cocktail 37
    chicken and tarragon
        salad 152
    egg curry 136
    jacket potato, chicken
        yogurt and mint
        filling 87
    minty cucumber salad
        179
    muesli 48
    peanut dip 64
    pitta pocket, tuna,
        cucumber and yogurt
        filling 89

Of further interest . . .

Healing Through Nutrition

A natural approach to treating 50 common illnesses with diet and nutrients

DR MELVYN R. WERBACH

This indispensable reference book provides the nutritional roots of and treatments for 50 common illnesses, from allergies and the common cold to cancer.

The world's authority on the relationship between nutrition and illness, Dr Melvyn Werbach makes it easy to learn what you can do to influence the course of your health via the nutrients that you feed your body. This highly accessible A–Z of nutritional health includes:

- an analysis of dietary factors affecting health and well-being
- a suggested healing diet for 50 common illnesses
- nutritional healing plans, with recommended dosages for vitamins, minerals and other essential nutrients
- an explanation of vitamin supplements and how they can improve your health

There are also guidelines on how to plan the right healing diet for yourself and how to diagnose food sensitivities. With this ground-breaking guide, you will be able to make informed decisions about the essential role of nutrients in your health and well-being.

The Good Calorie Diet

The revolutionary new fat-reducing diet plan

PHILIP LIPETZ

Pasta. The best way to fatten yourself up? It needn't be. It's a 'good' calorie – served with limited animal protein, it's an aid to fat reduction.

In *The Good Calorie Diet* Philip Lipetz explodes the traditional myths of weight loss and healthy diet. By showing how to identify and avoid high fat-forming foods, he demonstrates that by concentrating on healthy calories, appetites decrease, metabolism improves, cravings for those 'bad' calorie reverse and weight is *still* lost.

Foods which are high in natural sugar ('bad' calorie foods) increase the body's capacity to create fat – especially when eaten with other fat-forming foods. 'Good' calorie foods, on the other hand, decrease appetite, improve metabolism and reverse the 'bad' calorie cravings. By eating as much of the 'good' calorie foods as desired, cravings for 'bad' calories will be reduced and fat formation will be maintained at a low level.

Lipetz's book provides over 3,000 'good' calorie and 'bad' calorie foods, an easy-to-follow eating plan, mouthwatering menus, delicious and varied recipes, and useful tips for eating in and eating out.

HEALING THROUGH NUTRITION	0 7225 2941 4	£16.99	☐
THE GOOD CALORIE DIET	0 7225 3007 2	£4.99	☐
THE SUPREME VEGETARIAN COOKBOOK	0 7225 3113 3	£8.99	☐

All these books are available from your local bookseller or can be ordered direct from the publishers.

To order direct just tick the titles you want and fill in the form below:

Name: _____

Address: _____

_____

_____Postcode: _____

Send to: Thorsons Mail Order, Dept 3, HarperCollins*Publishers*, Westerhill Road, Bishopbriggs, Glasgow G64 2QT.
Please enclose a cheque or postal order or your authority to debit your Visa/Access account –

Credit card no: _____

Expiry date: _____

Signature: _____

– to the value of the cover price plus:
UK & BFPO: Add £1.00 for the first book and 25p for each additional book ordered.
Overseas orders including Eire: Please add £2.95 service charge. Books will be sent by surface mail but quotes for airmail despatches will be given on request.

24 HOUR TELEPHONE ORDERING SERVICE FOR ACCESS/VISA CARDHOLDERS – TEL: 0141 772 2281.